CLINICAL EVALUATION OF
THE NERVOUS SYSTEM

CLINICAL EVALUATION OF THE NERVOUS SYSTEM

JOHN F. SIMPSON, M.D.
Late Associate Professor of Neurology
The University of Michigan Medical School
Ann Arbor

KENNETH R. MAGEE, M.D.
Professor of Neurology
The University of Michigan Medical School
Ann Arbor

Little, Brown and Company
Boston

PREFACE

This text was written primarily for medical students. It originated in lectures and demonstrations prepared for first- and second-year students at the University of Michigan Medical School; a locally published version has been in use there for three years. Our goal has been to help the student understand the fundamentals of neurologic diagnosis. In discussing the neurologic history and examination we emphasize practical aspects of technique and interpretation. We do not go into detail about neurologic signs that are of interest to the specialist in neural sciences but are not necessary for the solution of most neurologic problems.

The first part of the book discusses the neurologic history and examination and how to interpret them; a guide to the localization of pathologic signs within the nervous system follows. The final section of the book describes diagnostic procedures such as lumbar puncture and a growing assemblage of radiologic techniques—pneumoencephalography, arteriography, electroencephalography, electromyography, and radioisotope scanning. Here the aim is to acquaint the student with the *nature* of these techniques, their indications and contraindications, and their value in clinical diagnosis. We do not attempt to describe these complex procedures in detail; for most medical students, to do so would be superfluous, and those who want to go further into the subject will require training beyond the basic curriculum.

A brief section on pediatric neurology is included even though many examination techniques and their interpretations apply to children as well as adults. Differences do occur, and they are of considerable importance in diagnosis.

This book is in no way intended to supplant any existing textbook on adult or pediatric neurology. It is offered purely as an introduction—an aid to basic understanding and perhaps a stimulus to further study. Classic methods of teaching neural sciences, with their intensive grounding in the basics followed much later by a cautious dip into clinical neurology, are everywhere being replaced by integrated or core-curriculum formats which blend the essentials with early exposure to actual clinical situations. In the light of this trend we tried, if not to simplify, at least to shape this complex subject in a manner that will enable students to grasp it readily. We hope they will find it a relatively comfortable way to develop initial skills.

During preparation of this new book we invited student and faculty criticism of the original version and, not surprisingly, were amply rewarded. Many of the comments from our Ann Arbor colleagues as well as those from physicians elsewhere were incorporated into the new version.

We are grateful to Mrs. Diane Culver for her assistance in typing the manuscript.

J. F. S.
K. R. M.

During the final preparation of this book, Dr. Simpson died in an automobile accident. I have lost a close friend and colleague. He was respected and admired by all who knew him, both as a physician and as an individual.

K. R. M.

CONTENTS

CLINICAL EVALUATION OF
THE NERVOUS SYSTEM

1 THE NEUROLOGIC HISTORY

Because the nervous system may be involved in many different disease processes, the neurologic evaluation is an integral part of the general medical examination. Some diseases that arise in other body systems have important neurologic aspects—for example, diabetes mellitus, hyperthyroidism and other endocrine disorders, collagen diseases, hypertension, uremia, cirrhosis, and certain types of anemia. Various therapeutic drugs in common use show side effects resulting from nervous system dysfunction; certain poisons exert similar effects. It is therefore essential that the initial history take note of such conditions.

The information required for the neurologic history consists of the patient's chief complaint (symptoms), details of his present illness, his past medical history and that of his family, and pertinent factors in his socioeconomic background. The format is traditional in all branches of medicine. Because of the close relation of neurology to general medicine, no aspect of the general medical evaluation can be eliminated when the patient's symptoms suggest a neurologic disorder.

THE CHIEF COMPLAINT

The physician must elicit the reason why the patient is consulting him at this point in time. The chief complaint is the symptom or symptom complex of most concern to the patient—*not* that which the physician may adjudge the most important. The complaint should be recorded in the patient's own words, if possible, rather than in medical jargon.

THE PRESENT ILLNESS

This portion of the history is a chronologic account of the development of the symptoms noted. At this stage the physician must be, above all, a good listener. It is important that he not constantly interrupt the patient's train of thought by asking too many specific questions or questions that lead to possible inaccuracies. The patient must be free to expand his thoughts naturally. Dates are important and should be included whenever the patient is reasonably sure of them. The account should also include the reasons for and the results of any previous hospitalizations and medical consultations, as well as opinions, therapy, diagnostic procedures, and any other events affecting his symptoms. If the patient tends to ramble or become lost in irrelevant details, the physician may have to redirect the conversation to ensure that important details will not be omitted. But in any event, this initial interview is the physician's opportunity to establish rapport with the patient and his family and to obtain a concise and accurate record of the illness.

While the patient is talking, the physician should note his behavior, attitude, and personal appearance, because these form an important part of the overall evaluation. Such observations can yield information regarding organic or functional mental disorders, the patient's insight into his condition and his ability to accept it, and the approach the physician should follow in discussing the diagnostic and therapeutic plans and the prognosis.

As the patient tells his story, he may mention certain symptoms that have special significance in relation to the nervous system. Sometimes these are specific—for example, a convulsion can arise only from direct involvement of the nervous system. More often, however, the symptoms described are not specific but may indicate either a neurologic disorder or a disease of some other system. Weakness of the arms and legs is a common neurologic complaint, but it is also common in other disorders such as thyroid disease, neoplasm, and infections. Complaints such as dizziness, tiredness, backache, headache, and blurred vision may stem from psychologic problems as well as from neurologic disease. It is only the synthesis of details obtained from a thorough history and from the physical examination that allows the physician to decide whether he is dealing with a neurologic problem, a neurologic complication of a general medical problem, or a psychosomatic disorder. Not infrequently, continued observation is necessary to arrive at the correct diagnosis.

When the patient's complete history has been obtained the physician should determine as precisely as possible the anatomic site of the symptoms and the nature of onset—sudden, rapid, or slow—as well as circumstances surrounding the onset: injuries, concurrent illness, contact with ill persons, a change or cessation of medications, or emotional problems. The course and duration of the present illness are noted, especially whether it has been intermittent, steadily progressive, or improving. When the illness is chronic, the physician should analyze the patient's reason for coming to him at this particular time. For example, another disorder may be developing intercurrently; or the patient may simply need more supportive care or is hoping for a new kind of treatment that will be more effective.

Certain nonspecific but important neurologic complaints are so common that if the patient does not mention them the physician should make it a point to ask about them. These major complaints include:

HEADACHE. It is important to record the location, character, duration, and frequency of the headache, as well as any factors which seem to either aggravate or relieve the pain.

DIZZINESS. Dizziness is a nonspecific term which means different things to different people but usually refers to a lightheaded sensation. From the medical standpoint, true vertigo contains a rotatory component—the patient's environment seems to whirl around him, or his body seems to rotate in relation to the environment. The relation to posture is important, that is, whether the dizziness is brought on by suddenly standing up or turning or bending. Other symptoms simplified by use of the term *dizziness* include brief alterations of consciousness, suggesting a convulsion or cerebrovascular insufficiency. *Dizziness* is sometimes used by patients to indicate unsteadiness in walking; if the meaning is not clear, it helps to ask the patient whether the dizziness seems to come from inside his head or from trouble in using his legs.

VISUAL DISTURBANCES. Decrease in vision, blurred vision, double vision, and other disturbances are common; as with headache, the character, duration, localization, and frequency must be determined.

BOWEL OR BLADDER DYSFUNCTION. Urinary bladder dysfunction, such as frequency, urgency, and incontinence, are important symptoms. Bowel disturbances are usually less significant in neurologic diagnosis, but complaints of constipation, diarrhea, or bowel incontinence should be noted.

WEAKNESS. The physician should determine whether the weakness is diffuse or localized, progressive or stationary, and whether it varies during the day and is associated with pain.

NUMBNESS. As with dizziness, the description of numbness varies from one person to another. Most often it implies loss of sensation or odd sensations in a specific body area, but some patients confuse it with weakness, incoordination, or faintness.

PAIN. Any complaint of pain should be evaluated as to location, nature, duration, variation with time, and relation to trauma or other conditions. The influence of body position or motion should be considered, as well as details of previous attempts to relieve the pain.

PAST MEDICAL HISTORY

An accurate account of all past illnesses and injuries should be obtained and recorded in chronologic order. The results of medical or surgical treatment should be reviewed, and any residual problems noted; also the ingestion of any medication on a long-term basis.

REVIEW OF SYSTEMS

Complaints referable to all organ systems should be recorded; information about symptoms important to the diagnosis may be brought out by careful questioning if the patient fails to mention them. The form and outline for the review of systems are the same for neurology as for the other specialties, except that neuromuscular complaints, usually recorded in the review of systems, should be specifically discussed in the present illness, whether or not such complaints are a part of the chief complaint.

SOCIAL HISTORY

The patient's cultural, social, and economic status must be evaluated since these often play a major role in plans for diagnostic and therapeutic procedures. The information to be recorded includes the patient's marital status and number and ages of his children, his work history and present employment, with special attention to exposure to toxic substances, and the extent of the patient's indulgence in alcohol, tobacco, and drugs. The financial drain imposed by chronic disease may be considerable; for this reason, the type of hospitalization and medical insurance, along with other potential sources of financial aid (family or community), should be part of the record.

FAMILY HISTORY

Many neurologic diseases are hereditary; therefore an accurate family history is essential and may provide the key to a diagnosis. Have any of the patient's blood relatives had a similar disorder? If the same type of illness has occurred among his immediate family, might it represent exposure to infection or chronic poisoning rather than a hereditary disorder? In addition to neurologic or other diseases, the notes on the family history should include instances of mental disorders and hospitalization in psychiatric facilities, for these may reveal organic brain disease that the patient's relatives have termed "nervous breakdown."

GENERAL CONSIDERATIONS

The importance of the art and skill of history taking can hardly be overemphasized. In neurology perhaps more than in other branches of medicine the medical history is often the crucial factor in the diagnosis. In fact, there are several important neurologic disorders in which the physical examination is entirely normal and the diagnosis rests on the history alone. This can happen, for example, in trigeminal neuralgia or migraine as well as in so-called idiopathic epilepsy. Sometimes the patient's illness is still incipient, its eventual course and direction uncertain; here the family history may serve to predict the localization of the disease within the nervous system and afford the opportunity for early specific treatment. And finally, the process of obtaining the history gives the physician his best opportunity to get to know the patient, understand his problems and worries, and through personal observation gain information that might otherwise be missed entirely.

2   THE NEUROLOGIC EXAMINATION

The neurologic examination yields data about the functional state of the nervous system and thus may provide objective evidence regarding the symptoms described by the patient. To evaluate this evidence from a diagnostic standpoint requires basic knowledge of the anatomy of the nervous system in relation to its specific functions.

Therefore the examination procedures are grouped according to functional units—particularly mental status, speech and language, cranial nerves, motor system, sensory system, and reflexes. As the examination proceeds, the findings are correlated with pertinent historical details, the other portions of the examination, and applicable anatomic and physiologic details. Often the results lead to accurate localization of the site of disease in the nervous system.

In the following sections of this chapter, procedures for the neurologic examination are discussed along with certain important anatomic features necessary for accurate interpretation of the results.

MENTAL STATUS

At the outset, the patient's mental status may suggest organic abnormalities, as distinguished from functional disorders such as psychoneurosis, which then guides the physician in planning subsequent studies. For the evaluation of mental status the history of the patient's signs and symptoms is of primary importance; it is essential to have information about his previous mental state. A *change* in behavior or mentality is especially significant—for example, slovenliness in a previously rigid and compulsive housewife, or withdrawn sullenness in a formerly extroverted salesman. Also, preexisting neurotic behavior patterns or personality disturbances may reappear or intensify with the onset of brain disease. Often it is necessary to obtain some or all of this information from relatives or friends of the patient.

In addition to changes in behavior, information should be sought regarding the patient's ability to reason, form judgments, plan ahead, and remember accurately. His age and educational background, of course, are related to his intellectual function. If his education is limited, he may not be able to solve arithmetic problems or give clear descriptions of current or past events. Similarly, the expression of abstract concepts may be difficult for him even though his native intelligence and reasoning ability may be normal.

Technique of Examination

Assessment of the level of consciousness is the first step. The average patient is alert and responsive; any deviations from this pattern may be significant. Evidence of indifference, drowsiness, lethargy, or deeper levels of unconsciousness such as stupor or coma should be examined in detail, chiefly through the patient's response to stimuli of various kinds.

Unusual behavior or appearance should be noted. For example, certain patients with organic mental deterioration become slovenly in personal care and dress. On the other hand, persons with functional psychoses may exhibit bizarre actions or make irrelevant comments. Such deviations should be carefully recorded though at this point in the examination they may not suggest any particular disease entity.

Orientation should next be considered. The patient should know where he is, who he is, and the date and time of day; he should also understand the situation he is in. The examiner should record his impression of the patient's emotional state—whether he is calm, anxious, fearful, belligerent, and so forth. Evidence of unusual thought trends should be noted; for example, preoccupation with certain body functions or abnormalities, or with the actions of other persons, may prove significant. These trends are seen in both functional and organic disorders of the central nervous system.

When the patient is able to cooperate with the examiner, an adequate intellectual assessment can usually be made in a brief period. Performance on specific intellectual tests should be evaluated.

MEMORY OF PAST EVENTS. The patient's memory of past events is assessed by asking him several straightforward questions about events in his own past, such as his birthday or year of graduation. Recent memory can be tested by giving the patient two or three common objects to remember and then asking him to name them after five or ten minutes. Immediate recall, another form of memory, is best tested by repeating a series of single digits and asking the patient to repeat them. Normally a person can repeat at least six digits, and many people can repeat eight or nine.

ARITHMETIC ABILITY. Following memory assessment, arithmetic ability is evaluated, usually by having the patient subtract 7 from 100 with subsequent subtractions of 7 from each remainder. Other appropriate tests can be devised by the examiner, according to the educational level and capabilities of the patient.

GENERAL KNOWLEDGE. General knowledge can be tested by asking the patient to name several presidents (if he is from the United States) from the present backward or to give some familiar capital cities, directions to major local cities, or important current events.

ABILITY TO COMPREHEND ABSTRACT RELATIONSHIPS. Important information may be obtained by testing the patient's ability to comprehend abstract relationships. One way to do this is to quote a common proverb such as "a bird in the hand is worth two in the bush" and then ask the patient to explain what is meant. Patients with organic mental impairment and also certain schizophrenic patients may give a concrete answer, failing to recognize the abstract principle involved.

Should this brief screening uncover only equivocal evidence of mental impairment, additional psychologic studies should be obtained.

Clinicopathologic Correlations

Although intellectual functions within the brain cannot be completely compartmentalized in terms of cerebral localization, certain general-

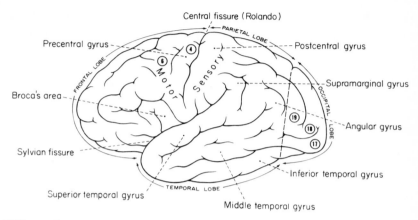

FIG. 1. Lateral view of the left cerebral hemisphere. Broca's area is related to vocal expression of language. Portions of the superior temporal, supramarginal, and angular gyri are important in the reception of language.

izations can be made. The ability to conceptualize, abstract, plan ahead, and formulate rational judgments of problems or events is largely a function of the *frontal lobes* (Figs. 1–3; see also Chapter **3**, "The Cerebral Hemispheres"), particularly the anterior portions. Significant disease in these regions, affecting either one or both sides, may cause a breakdown in the person's relationship to his environment and is manifested by inattention to grooming, appearance, and personal habits. It will also impair his judgment and the making of

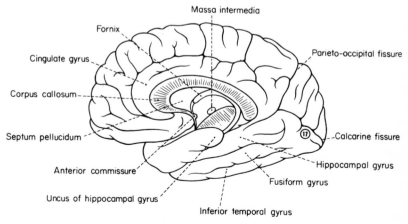

FIG. 2.   Medial view of the right cerebral hemisphere.

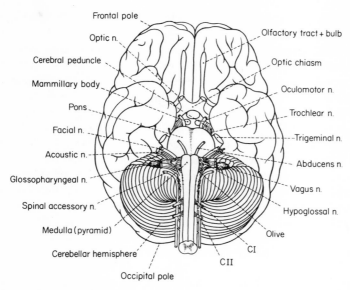

Frontal pole

Optic n.

Cerebral peduncle

Mammillary body

Pons

Facial n.

Acoustic n.

Glossopharyngeal n.

Spinal accessory n.

Medulla (pyramid)

Cerebellar hemisphere

Occipital pole

Olfactory tract + bulb

Optic chiasm

Oculomotor n.

Trochlear n.

Trigeminal n.

Abducens n.

Vagus n.

Hypoglossal n.

Olive

C I

C II

FIG. 3. Basal view of the brain.

decisions and plans, interfering with his occupation or management of the household. These persons tend to become preoccupied with themselves, suspicious of others, rigid, and difficult to influence. Higher intellectual functions involving abstractions and reasoning are also impaired.

Memories are generally thought to be formed and stored in certain regions of the *temporal lobes,* which have intimate connections with most other portions of the cortex, including the frontal lobes. In organic disease, the patient's memories for recent events and immediate recall are impaired much more severely than are memories of the remote past. It is not uncommon for a person to be able to name his grade school and some of his grade school teachers, a childhood address, and names of brothers and sisters, but be unable to state what he had for lunch that day or what the examiner's name is, or to repeat more than three or four numbers given to him verbally.

Lesions of the *parietal lobe,* especially if bilateral, may produce severe impairment of perceptual functions, including lack of appreciation of the environment and inability to interpret visual stimuli. Such patients may have great difficulty in communication and in understanding what goes on around them.

The degree of impairment of mental function caused by a given lesion depends not only on its location but also on its speed of development and growth. For example, a large frontal lobe tumor may produce only mild impairment if the tumor grows slowly. Conversely, a smaller lesion with rapid onset and growth, associated with edema and hemorrhage, will produce much more profound impairment.

The precise localization of a lesion causing mental symptoms depends on the detection of associated neurologic findings. For example, absence of the sense of smell accompanying an organic mental syndrome suggests a lesion in the inferior portion of the frontal lobe, since the olfactory pathways are in this region. The finding of hemiparesis suggests a lesion in the more posterior portion of the frontal lobe. In the absence of such associated neurologic abnormalities, certain laboratory evaluations are usually necessary to localize the lesion causing mental impairment.

SPEECH AND LANGUAGE

Speech is a complex function involving the most intimate interrelationship of numerous areas of the brain, peripheral nervous system, the muscles concerned with speech, and the larynx.

Speech disorders important in neurologic diagnosis can be divided into three general groups: dysarthria, dysphonia, and aphasia. Lisping—the omission, distortion, or substitution of consonants—and stammering, manifested by pauses in speech flow together with repeated attempts to produce a sound, are not associated with the neurologic disorders of speech that are considered here.

Dysarthria

Dysarthria is a general term indicating defects in articulation, enunciation, and rhythm of speech. It usually results from impairment of the musculature of tongue, palate, pharynx, or lips because of incoordination, weakness, abnormal innervation, or such extraneural problems as poorly fitting dentures and malformations of the oral structures. It is characterized by slurring, slowness, indistinctness, and breaks in normal speech rhythm. A common example of dysarthric speech is that of a drunk, in whom alcohol has altered the centers in the brainstem and cerebellum concerned with coordination of speech musculature.

Dysarthria is usually detectable in ordinary conversation with the patient. It can be confirmed by having the patient repeat a difficult test phrase such as "Methodist Episcopal" or "third riding artillery brigade." Examination of those structures concerned with normal speech production often reveal other neurologic abnormalities, and these findings offer important clues to the cause of the dysarthria. For example, in the dysarthria caused by weakness of the muscles (tongue, palate, pharynx, or jaw), the patient's speech is generally of reduced volume and nasal because of palatal weakness and inability to close the nasopharynx. It is usually slow and laborious. The causes for such weakness are not numerous; they include amyotrophic lateral sclerosis, which affects the bulbar cranial nerve nuclei, and pseudobulbar palsy, myasthenia gravis, and certain primary muscle diseases.

Dysphonia

Dysphonia is a disorder of vocalization characterized by the abnormal production of sounds from the larynx. Various abnormalities of the larynx itself or of its innervation are the usual causes of dysphonia. The primary complaint is hoarseness, ranging from mild roughness of the voice to inability to produce laryngeal sound. Whispered voice sounds are intact in dysphonia unless associated with dysarthria. The examiner and patient are usually aware of hoarseness, but in doubtful cases, abnormalities of laryngeal function can often be brought out by having the patient say "E" to produce strong adduction of the vocal cords. If the cords are not functioning normally, hoarseness or roughness will be evident. In all questionable cases, inspection of the vocal cords with a laryngeal mirror (indirect laryngoscopy) should be performed. Also, the functions of the vagus nerve should be carefully evaluated, since this nerve innervates the laryngeal muscles.

The many causes of dysphonia include a considerable number which are not neurologic; for example, laryngitis or tumors of the vocal cord. Among the important neurologic causes are injuries to the recurrent laryngeal nerve from thyroid surgery, tumors in the region of the jugular foramen, infarction of the lateral portion of the medulla (occlusion of the posterior inferior cerebellar or vertebral artery), and tumors of the brainstem.

Aphasia

Aphasia denotes the inability to use and understand written and spoken words (language symbols) as a result of disorders of cortical centers for speech or of their interconnections in the dominant cerebral hemisphere, the peripheral mechanisms for speech remaining intact. As thus defined, aphasia excludes dysarthria and dysphonia and also may exclude instances in which the patient, for one reason or another, is confused or shows signs of generally depressed brain function.

Aphasia may be detected in ordinary conversation with a patient. If he relates a long and complex history with consistently appropriate word choice and syntax, responds promptly to questions and requests, and demonstrates the ability to read and understand, the presence of aphasia is unlikely. Nevertheless, if the history suggests the possibility of a lesion in areas concerned with speech, formal evaluation of written and spoken language functions is advisable. In such instances, however, any disturbance in speech or language usually is obvious.

The major difficulty for the examiner is to distinguish between a true language disturbance (aphasia) and other disorders such as dysarthria, confusion, and mutism. It is important to keep in mind that if a patient's speech can be transcribed into logical sentences, or if he can express himself normally in writing, he is probably not aphasic, even if his speech is markedly dysarthric and almost unintelligible. Similarly, if a patient appears totally mute but can express himself correctly in writing and gestures, he is not aphasic.

Aphasia has been classified in many ways, not all of which are clinically important; they reflect the great interest and importance of aphasia from psychologic, as well as neurologic, viewpoints. A current concept of aphasia encompasses two major subdivisions: *nonfluent* and *fluent* aphasia. In nonfluent aphasia the patient utters little or no speech, either spontaneously or in reply to questions. If words are produced, it is with great effort, and they are spoken very slowly and with poor articulation. In some cases, one or two words or sounds, often expletives, constitute the entire speech output. In this variety of aphasia, therefore, the expression of the patient's thoughts is severely impaired by his inability to produce words, but his understanding of spoken and written language is intact or nearly so. Therefore in some classifications this type of aphasia is termed *expressive*. *Agraphia* denotes a similar problem in expressing thoughts in writing.

Fluent aphasia, the other major subdivision, is characterized by normal or even increased production of well-articulated words, many times in long phrases and sentences, but with defects in the thought content and errors in words used. The use of incorrect words, for example "bat" for "ball," and mispronunciation of words, are frequent. This type of word production is termed *paraphasia*. Neologisms, words with no meaning whatever, also occur. The overall effect in severe cases may be incomprehensible jargon. In addition, many patients with this variety of aphasia fail to comprehend written or spoken requests and are unable to repeat phrases they hear. Because of impaired comprehension of requests, either written or spoken, the term *receptive* has been used for this type of aphasia.

If aphasia testing is indicated, a relatively simple scheme can be used as a guide to a systematic analysis:

1. Vocal expression
   a. Observe the number of words which the patient uses; is the word supply adequate for complete sentences?
   b. Does the patient use only one or two words, or a phrase or two, continually, with little or no other understandable speech?
   c. Does it seem that the patient is comprehending your requests but is having great difficulty in expressing his thoughts?
2. Written expression
   a. Ask the patient to write his name and address and a common sentence.
   b. Ask him to copy a sentence from a newspaper or a magazine.
3. Comprehension of spoken language
   a. Give a series of spoken requests of increasing complexity and note whether the patient carries them out correctly.
   b. Ask the patient to repeat several sentences after you.
   c. Ask the patient to pick out some common objects from a group.
4. Comprehension of written language
   a. Give a series of written or printed requests to the patient and observe him for signs of recognition and understanding. Be sure to avoid verbal or gesture clues.
   b. Place a group of common objects in front of the patient, then show him the written names for some of them and observe whether he can match these to the correct objects.
5. Communication by gesture—for example, shrugging the shoulders and shaking the head—may occur if speech is absent. Such communication should be noted, particularly as it indicates comprehension and an effort to respond appropriately.

In using this scheme of testing, you must be certain that vision and hearing are normal. Responses to several test items may be observed concurrently. Comprehension, of course, is essential for carrying out any type of instruction and should be observed throughout the examination. Bearing in mind the distinction between nonfluent and fluent aphasia, types of difficulty in expression must be distinguished. In fluent aphasia, for example, profuse production of words may occur with paraphasia, jargon, and substitutions, and there may be a severe associated defect in comprehension of spoken language. An analogous problem in expression of written language occurs in fluent aphasia, marked by the writing of meaningless words and inability to comprehend written language.

Aphasia has been the subject of a vast amount of research and innumerable publications. Over the years many attempts have been made to subclassify aphasia and to localize specific kinds of aphasia to specific areas of cerebral cortex. However, aphasia does not lend itself to simplistic and rigid subclassifications based on specific cortical areas, and most aphasia contains elements of receptive and expressive difficulties.

As indicated earlier, the physician must be cautious about making a diagnosis of aphasia in the presence of confusion or obtundation, mechanical impairment of speech production such as incoordination or paresis of speech musculature, or simply lack of cooperation. Patients who have extensive intracerebral lesions of any kind are often obtunded and confused regardless of the location of the lesion whether the lesion is a single mass or a widespread metabolic derangement. In such patients. specific analysis of language function is difficult, and one cannot assume that the lack of ability to understand a request, name an object, or express a thought is necessarily a specific aphasic defect. The patient must have a clear sensorium and be relatively calm and cooperative to establish the existence of true aphasia.

Aphasia usually indicates a lesion that is localized to the left cerebral hemisphere. The left hemisphere is dominant for speech in the right-handed population and in the majority of the left-handed population. In perhaps 20% of left-handed persons, speech functions are largely localized to the right cerebral hemisphere and in a small percentage of persons, mostly left-handed, there appears to be bilateral representation of speech.

The lesion may be further localized within the left hemisphere according to the variety of aphasia. Nonfluent aphasia is produced by a lesion in the lateral inferior portion of the frontal lobe (Broca's area; see Fig. 1) on the dominant side. Since this area is adjacent to the motor cortex and its projections, hemiparesis is commonly found on the right side. If the aphasia is of a fluent variety, the lesion is in the left temporal and parietal lobes; many patients with this type of aphasia also have hemiparesis. If there is no hemiparesis but the patient simply shows a language pattern of jargon, paraphasia, incorrect word usage, and lack of comprehension, there may be some difficulty in differentiating this picture from that of psychosis. Aphasia is usually of abrupt onset, resulting from cerebrovascular occlusion or head trauma, and only coincidentally occurs in patients with emotional problems.

If the aphasia is a nonfluent variety, with the patient showing not only great difficulty in expressing his thoughts but also marked loss of comprehension, it is termed *global aphasia,* implying a larger lesion involving both Broca's area and the temporoparietal speech regions. Such patients have hemiparesis on the opposite side.

By far the most common cause of aphasia is cerebrovascular disease involving the distribution of the middle cerebral artery, which supplies most of the cortical areas for speech and language (these areas are indicated in Fig. 1). Other causes include trauma, tumor, abscess, intracerebral hemorrhage, and subdural hematoma.

Agnosia and Apraxia

AGNOSIA. Agnosia is defined as the inability to recognize objects or symbols by means of the senses—hearing, sight, or touch—the primary receptors remaining intact. For example, impaired recognition of objects by sight is termed *visual agnosia;* impaired recognition of common sounds is *auditory agnosia.* In this sense agnosia differs from aphasia, which specifically concerns language symbols.

The anatomic relationship between the areas integrating higher level visual and auditory perception with language areas is so close that the differentiation of agnosia from aphasia is not crucial from a practical clinical standpoint. Mixtures of agnostic and aphasic difficulties are common. Although agnosia results from a lesion of the dominant hemisphere, as does aphasia, there is an exception in that defective recognition of objects by touch (tactile agnosia) develops in the extremity contralateral to the side of the lesion (parietal lobe). Such a defect is usually called *astereognosis* (see p. 73) rather than tactile agnosia.

The term *anosognosia* means lack of awareness or denial of existence of his disease by the patient; *autotopagnosia* means a disturbance in recognition of body parts. These disorders relate to one's awareness of one's body in relation to the environment, and their symptoms occur contralateral to the involved parietal lobe. For example, a hemiplegic patient with this type of cortical sensory dysfunction may completely deny the presence of paralysis on one side. Such disturbances are usually most easily detected in lesions of the minor hemisphere, probably because aphasic defects in the dominant hemisphere prevent the patient's expression of these denial phenomena.

APRAXIA.   Apraxia is a concept of important theoretical and lesser practical interest. It is defined as the inability to carry out a purposeful movement when comprehension is intact, despite the absence of paralysis, ataxia, or sensory disturbances that would interfere with performance of the movement. For example, in apraxia of the arm, the patient, if offered a comb, cannot demonstrate how it is used. A subconscious movement, such as scratching the head, is performed normally. Similarly, he may not be able to execute a simple command like striking a match. Apraxia of gait and speech and of any type of motor activity may occur.

Apraxia is not strictly localizable, for it may result from lesions in the dominant or nondominant hemisphere, or both hemispheres. Constructional apraxia—the inability to draw or express forms, especially three-dimensional structures—and apraxia for dressing are detected most commonly with lesions of the nondominant parietal lobe and are related to disturbances in spatial awareness.

The importance of apraxia lies in what it may signify, rather than in its precise localizing value. To cite an example: A middle-aged man became depressed and complained of difficulty in walking for a two-month period. There were no positive findings except apraxia of gait and mental depression. A diagnosis of hysterical paralysis was considered before studies led to the correct diagnosis of bilateral subdural hematoma subsequently successfully treated.

THE CRANIAL NERVES

OLFACTORY NERVE (CRANIAL NERVE I)

The paired olfactory nerves mediate the sense of smell. Smell bears a complimentary relation to the appreciation of taste; therefore, either the absence (anosmia) or decrease in sensitivity (hyposmia) of the sense of smell is commonly associated with the complaint of loss of taste, even though specific tests may show the taste sense to be intact.

Technique of Examination

Common, mildly aromatic substances such as vanilla, cloves, or coffee are best used for the olfactory test. With the patient's eyes closed, occlude one nostril and bring a vial of the substance near the open nostril. Ask the patient to indicate whether he smells something and to identify it. The sensing of odor is more important than its identification, for many patients have difficulty identifying substances under these conditions. The process is then repeated for the other nostril. Differences in perception and identification between the two sides may be important. Irritating substances such as ammonia should not be used, because these activate receptors from the trigeminal nerve and induce a sensory perception other than smell. Other substances such as tobacco or perfumed soap can be used if the examiner does not have a smell-test kit available.

Clinicoanatomic Correlations

The first cranial nerve actually consists of many tiny nerve filaments passing from the superior portion of the nasal cavity through the cribriform plate into the anterior cranial fossa (Fig. 4). Here they synapse in the olfactory bulb with cell bodies of neurons whose axons pass in the olfactory tracts to the region of the olfactory trigone, where complex bilateral central connections occur.

The most common causes of decreased smell are not specifically neurogenic but rather are related to nasal disorders, for example, those resulting from allergic rhinitis, upper respiratory infection, and heavy cigarette smoking. Lesions of the tracts are uncommon. Occasionally, however, a tumor may originate in the region of the olfactory tract (usually an olfactory groove meningioma), causing unilateral or bilateral anosmia. Anosmia may occur as a sequel to meningitis or subarachnoid hemorrhage, or as the result of head injury damaging

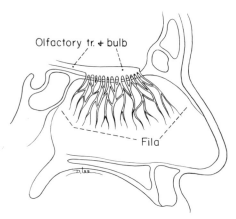

Olfactory tr. + bulb

Fila

FIG. 4. Olfactory nerve, illustrating distribution of filaments within the nose and the olfactory bulb and tract (*tr.*) within the anterior cranial fossa.

the olfactory nerve filaments as they pass through the cribriform plate.

Hallucinations of smell may occur with lesions in parts of the brain associated with the appreciation of smell (usually in the temporal lobes) but are not directly related to the first cranial nerve itself. In lesions of the central olfactory pathway beyond the olfactory tract the primary perception of odors remains intact.

OPTIC NERVE (CRANIAL NERVE II)

The optic nerves carry visual impulses from the retina of the eye to the optic chiasm, and from this point the impulses enter other visual pathways leading to various areas of the cerebral cortex for recognition and interpretation of visual images. Other fibers of the optic nerve take part in ocular reflexes. The visual system is illustrated in Figure 5. In studying the function of the optic nerves, the entire visual system is actually studied. Because of its extent and its intimate relations with other areas, much valuable information can be obtained from careful study of this system.

Clinicoanatomic Correlations

Visual field defects are extremely important in determining the anatomic location of the causative lesion. The visual pathways are extensive, and lesions giving rise to disorders in vision may occur anywhere from the eye itself to the occipital cortex. Figure 5 shows the anatomic sites of common lesions corresponding to the visual field defects

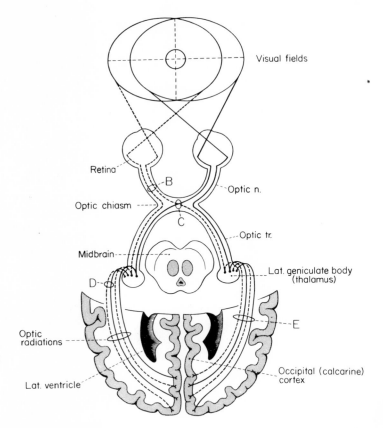

FIG. 5. The visual system. Lesions at *B, C, D*, and *E* correspond to visual field defects B, C, D, and E in Figure 6.

shown in Figure 6. In general, reduced visual acuity is caused by a disease involving the eye, the optic nerve, or the optic chiasm. When the site of disease is posterior to the optic chiasm, some macular vision remains and the visual loss may not be significant even though peripheral visual field defects may be large.

The following principles govern the evaluation of defects in the visual field.

1. A lesion in the nasal side of the retina or in optic nerve fibers subserving it causes a defect in the temporal half of the visual field for that eye. The reverse applies to the temporal retina. A lesion in or central to the inferior part of the retina causes a defect in the

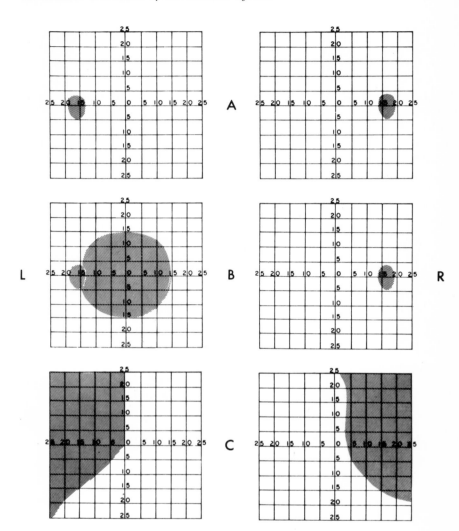

FIG. 6. Visual fields (by tangent screen). (A) normal; (B) scotoma, left eye; (C) bitemporal hemianopia; (D) right superior homonymous quadrantanopia; (E) left homonymous hemianopia with sparing of the macula; (F) spiral field, left eye.

superior half of the visual field. The reverse applies to the superior retina.

2. A lesion in the retina or in one optic nerve causes a visual field defect in that eye; in the opposite eye the field is normal. The most

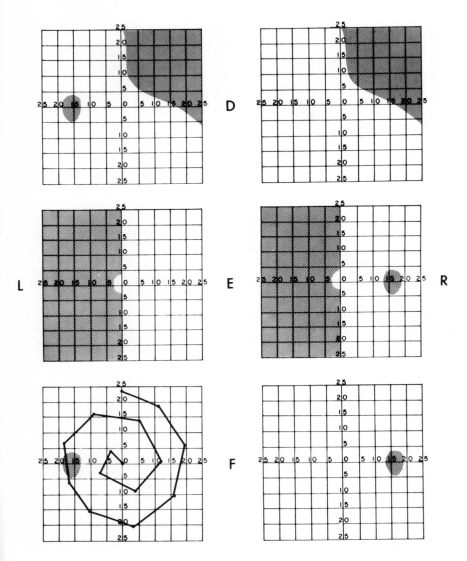

common defect resulting from lesions in this location is a *scotoma,* an island of decreased or absent vision within an otherwise normal field. A normal scotoma, called the *physiologic blind spot,* results from the absence of visual receptor cells on the discs. The spot normally measures 5 to 8 degrees, but may enlarge as papilledema develops.

3. A lesion of the optic chiasm leads to *bitemporal hemianopia,*

the loss of the temporal portions of the visual field of both eyes, resulting from interruption of the crossing fibers from the nasal sides of the retinas.

4. Lesions posterior to the chiasm, in the *optic tract* and *optic radiations,* cause homonymous defects; the defect occurs in corresponding halves of the fields in both eyes, occupying either the right or the left half of the total visual field. For example, the nasal field may be affected in the right eye and the temporal field in the left, resulting in left homonymous hemianopia. The anatomic basis for this effect is the juxtaposition of fibers from both retinas in the optic tracts and radiations.

5. A lesion in the parietal lobe may interrupt pathways carrying visual impulses from the superior portion of the retina since these fibers remain superior when they fan out in the optic radiations. The result is a homonymous defect in the inferior quadrant of the visual field (inferior quandrantanopia).

6. Lesions limited to the temporal lobe may interrupt pathways from the inferior portion of the retina, which remain inferior as they traverse the temporal lobes, and the result is a homonymous defect in the superior quadrants (superior quadrantanopia). The quadrantic homonymous defects are not common; usually there is homonymous hemianopia which is complete or nearly complete. In some instances the macular area is spared, particularly with the more posterior lesions in the optic radiations. The reason for this is not well established, and the point is of limited value in diagnostic studies.

Diseases that produce scotomas include glaucoma, retinal artery occlusion, and inflammation of the optic nerve or optic disc (*optic* or *retrobulbar neuritis*). Of the lesions at or above the optic chiasm which result in *bitemporal* field defects, the most important are such tumors as pituitary adenoma and craniopharyngioma. *Homonymous hemianopia* is usually caused by cerebral infarction resulting from vascular occlusion, as well as from brain tumor, injury, and abscess. Visual field defects other than those described here may be encountered, but in most cases the anatomic site of the related lesion may be detected if the examiner is thoroughly familiar with the basic relationships illustrated in Figures 5 and 6.

It should be noted that visual field defects have been observed in connection with mental and emotional disturbances. Here the differential diagnosis is suggested by the appearance of peripheral constriction of the entire visual field, producing "tubular" or "gunbarrel" vision. In contrast to the constriction resulting from an anatomic lesion, the size of the constricted field in an emotional disorder remains the same whether the patient is close to or at some distance from the examiner or the tangent screen. As testing proceeds, the field may continue to constrict as its margins are mapped out, and as a result it becomes smaller and smaller, producing "spiral" fields (see Fig. 6).

Technique of Examination

Two aspects of vision are commonly tested: visual acuity and the visual fields. Visual acuity is the ability of the eye to perceive fine detail, as in reading or in perceiving small objects, and is subserved by the *macula*, a very small area located in the center of the retina and composed of specialized cells called *cones*. The peripheral portions of the retina are primarily composed of less specialized cells called *rods*.

The visual fields constitute the peripheral limits of vision and all visual function within their limits. The visual fields are studied, therefore, by delineating these peripheral limits and also by searching for areas within the limits where vision is absent.

In addition to these two types of visual testing, examination of the optic nerve also includes a study of the retina and the optic discs with the ophthalmoscope.

VISUAL ACUITY. Visual acuity is usually tested by the use of a card with printed sentences in various sizes of type (Jaeger types, after the inventor of this system). A wall chart (Snellen chart) for testing distance vision is satisfactory but less convenient. If the examiner does not have a standard card, ordinary newsprint (usually Jaeger 7) is satisfactory for a screening evaluation. Since refractive errors—those abnormalities of the refractive media of the eyeball causing imperfect focusing on the retina—are not usually important for neurologic diagnosis, visual acuity is tested with the patient wearing his glasses. Ask the patient to read a sentence or two with each eye separately, and note the smallest size type he can read. Visual acuity should be recorded in quantitative terms, such as Jaeger 7, in order to furnish a base line for future comparison. If a patient appears to have difficulty focusing his eyes, or holds the test card either far away or very close, he may have an undetected refractive error (farsightedness, nearsightedness, or astigmatism) and his visual acuity will not be an accurate indication of function in the visual neural pathways. In such instances, ophthalmologic consultation should be obtained.

VISUAL FIELDS. For screening purposes, the visual fields are examined by the method of *confrontation* (Fig. 7). Each eye is evaluated separately by covering the other eye. A control is established if the examiner closes his right eye, for example, when the patient's right eye is being examined. Thus, the examiner can compare the field of vision of his (normal) left eye with that of the patient's right eye. The four quadrants of the visual field should be evaluated by bringing a wiggling finger in from the periphery, equidistant from examiner and patient, until the patient indicates that he sees it, thus determining the peripheral limits in that quadrant. If a defect in the visual field of either eye is detected by this method, the configuration of the defect should be determined by moving the finger in from several areas within each affected quadrant. Since scotomas are often symptomatic, the patient may be able to describe the area involved. Such areas are carefully explored by moving a small object, such as a pin with a white head, from the center of the defect outward in all directions until its limits are reached. A sketch of any visual field defect should be made on the patient's record.

Examination of visual fields by the method of double simultaneous testing may provide additional information when tests with single stimuli are normal. With lesions of the visual association areas in the cortex (*not* the primary visual pathway), the patient may appre-

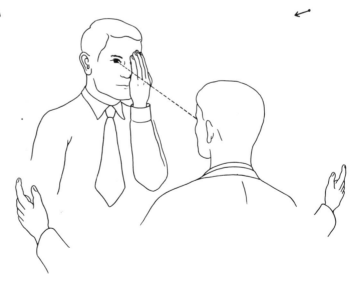

FIG. 7. Technique of confrontation. The *arrows* indicate the two other quadrants tested routinely. Each eye is tested separately.

ciate single stimuli normally but will fail to detect stimuli in the field opposite the lesion when both visual fields are tested at the same time. The method of testing is simple. Two stimuli, usually moving fingers, are presented simultaneously within the left and right visual fields and the patient is asked to state which finger is moving. Normally people state "both" with no hesitation. The detection of simultaneous stimuli relates to body imagery, which is discussed later in relation to cortical sensory perception (see p. 73). As the visual association areas are adjacent to the primary cortical center for visual reception, detection of a defect by simultaneous stimuli has the same importance in cerebral localization, from a practical clinical standpoint, as does detection of a defect causing a homonymous hemianopia.

More detailed study of visual field defects is accomplished by the use of a *perimeter,* in which the peripheral margins of the field are evaluated, and by a *tangent screen* examination, in which the central 25 degrees of the visual fields are evaluated in detail.

Optic Disc and Retina

The appearance of the optic disc, the anterior end of the optic nerve, and the surface of the retina is important in both neurologic and general medical diagnosis. The two most significant abnormalities of the optic discs are *papilledema* (choked disc) and *optic atrophy.* Papilledema (Fig. 8) is a swelling of the optic disc usually associated with increased intracranial pressure, regardless of cause.

The signs are subtle in the early stages of papilledema. Normally the retinal veins in the region of the disc pulsate spontaneously, and the absence of such pulsations may be the first sign. Another early sign is engorgement and relative increase in size of the retinal veins compared to the arterioles. As papilledema progresses, it is characterized by (1) indistinctness of the margin of the disc, (2) elevation of the disc above the surface of the retina, (3) disappearance of the normal cupping or concavity in the center of the disc, (4) arching and elevation of veins and arteries as they pass over the margin of the disc, and (5) enlargement of the physiologic blind spot (see below). In severe papilledema there may be hemorrhages within the disc and in the surrounding retina.

In spite of the presence of papilledema, visual acuity remains relatively normal for a time. Eventually, however, optic atrophy with blindness results unless the pressure is relieved. Thus, papilledema requires prompt evaluation and treatment.

Optic atrophy (Fig. 9) may be either primary or secondary. The

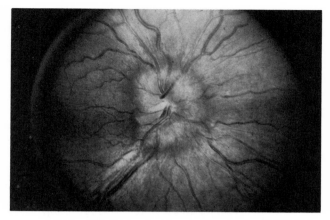

FIG. 8. Optic fundus, the disc showing moderate papilledema. Note the elevated margin and the venous engorgement.

primary type results from diseases affecting the optic nerve—for example, injury, compression by a tumor, or syphilis. The disc is pale lemon-yellow or white rather than the normal pinkish hue; the margin is very sharp and the physiologic cup may be accentuated. *Secondary* optic atrophy results from papilledema secondary to chronic increased intracranial pressure, and the disc has a grayish appearance and indistinct margins. Secondary optic atrophy is not pertinent to initial neurologic diagnosis. The diagnosis of papilledema

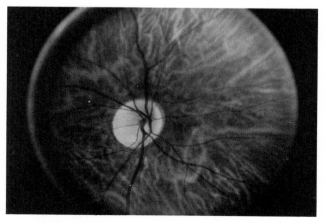

FIG. 9. Optic fundus, the disc showing primary optic atrophy. Note the flat, pale appearance of the disc.

and its cause is usually established and treatment rendered before this complication develops.

A careful ophthalmologic examination of structures visible in the retina is also important for both neurologic and general medical diagnosis. Disc changes are observed in patients with the most common neurologic problems—tumors, infections, trauma—but retinal abnormalities may be the key to diagnosis of some other primary neurologic disorders. Examples include lipid storage diseases of infancy, degenerative changes associated with neurologic disorders, and certain infections that may affect the central nervous system as well as the retina. These conditions are rare, however, and the most common and important retinal changes are those associated with systemic diseases that may have neurologic manifestations. These include exudates, hemorrhages, and arterial and venous abnormalities associated with diabetes, hypertension, and hematologic abnormalities.

OCULOMOTOR, TROCHLEAR, AND ABDUCENS NERVES (CRANIAL NERVES III, IV, AND VI)

These three nerves have similar functions which are customarily examined as a group. They act together (*conjugate function*) in controlling the ocular muscles to ensure that the eyes will remain parallel throughout their range of motion, thus maintaining binocular vision

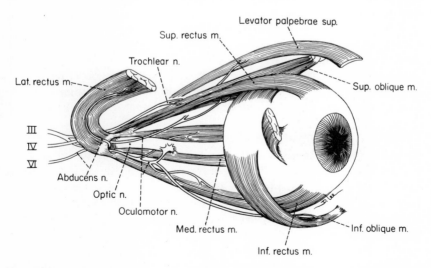

FIG. 10. Lateral view of right eyeball, illustrating the extraocular muscles with their nerves.

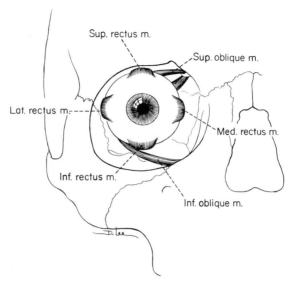

Sup. rectus m.

Sup. oblique m.

Lat. rectus m.

Med. rectus m.

Inf. rectus m.

Inf. oblique m.

D. Lee

FIG. 11.   Frontal view of right eyeball, illustrating the extraocular muscles.

(Figs. 10, 11). In addition, the oculomotor nerve controls the muscle (levator palpebrae superioris) which elevates the upper eyelid, and innervates the constrictor muscle of the pupil, which alters the pupil size in response to varying degrees of illumination or to convergence and accommodation.

A lesion affecting one or more of these nerves results in weakness of the corresponding muscles and consequent deviation of the eyeball from parallel, manifested by *diplopia* (double vision) or, if long-standing and especially in childhood, by suppression of vision in the affected eye. Drooping of the upper lid (ptosis) and sustained dilatation of the pupil may also result if the oculomotor nerve is affected.

Technique of Examination

To examine the function of these nerves, first inspect the eyes. Note the relative position of the upper eyelids with the patient gazing directly at you. When ptosis is sufficient to occlude vision in one or both eyes, the patient contracts the muscles of the forehead in an effort to lift the upper lid. (Sagging of the lower lid on one side may indicate weakness of the orbicularis oculi muscle, which is innervated by the seventh cranial nerve.)

Inspect the pupils in subdued light. They should appear round and approximately equal in size; however, since unequal pupils are found in about one-fourth of the normal population, this finding may not be significant, especially when the difference is small (1 mm.) and the pupillary reflexes are not impaired. Be certain that the patient has not had any medication instilled in the eye for purposes of constricting or dilating the pupil, since alterations in pupillary size or reactions are then of no diagnostic significance.

Next, evaluate the pupillary light reflex. Shine a bright light into one eye and observe the response of the pupils. Both pupils should constrict promptly when the light shines into one eye. The response of the pupil of the eye tested is called the *direct light reflex* and that of the pupil on the opposite side, the *consensual light reflex*. The reflex is especially brisk during youth and in persons with blue eyes.

Loss of the direct light reflex may result from disorders of the optic or oculomotor nerve on that side. Loss of the consensual light reflex may be due to lesions of either the optic nerve on the side tested or of the oculomotor nerve on the opposite side. Failure of pupillary reaction to light is most important as a sign of lesions in the oculomotor nerves or their connections. Disease of the optic nerve will also reduce or abolish the light reflex, but this is of less diagnostic importance because severe visual loss is obvious.

When a person gazes into the distance, the pupils become relatively dilated and the axes of the eyes are parallel. If the person then looks quickly at an object 6 to 8 inches from his face, both eyes adduct (turn medially), the pupils constrict, and the lenses become thicker because of relaxation of the suspensory ligament of the lens. These phenomena together constitute the *accommodation-convergence reflex*. Normally, adduction of the eyes and constriction of the pupils are easily seen, particularly in young individuals. Loss of this normal response may result from lesions of the third cranial nerves or their connections in the midbrain. Although the reflex is significant in optic function, it is not of major importance in neurologic diagnosis.

An associated pupillary reflex, the *ciliospinal reflex*, consists of dilatation of the ipsilateral pupil when the skin of the neck is pinched vigorously. The reflex is mediated through cervical sympathetic pathways and demonstrates their integrity.

To examine the extraocular muscles, the examiner should observe the visual axes—that is, the alignment of the two eyes with respect to each other. Deviation (lack of parallelism) of the axes is termed *strabismus* (or squint) and indicates weakness of one or more of the extraocular muscles, or lack of perfect neural coordination. After noting any obvious abnormalities of visual alignment as the patient looks straight ahead, the examiner evaluates extraocular muscle function in

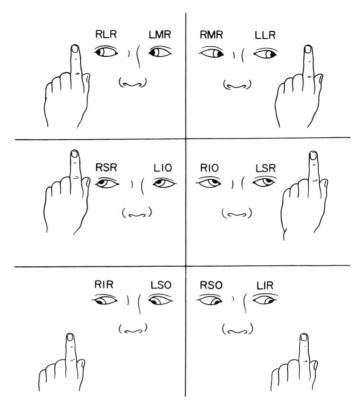

FIG. 12. Examination of extraocular muscles. Note that two muscles are involved (one yoke) in each cardinal direction of gaze. (*R* = right; *L* = left; *LR* = lateral rectus; *MR* = medial rectus; *SR* = superior rectus; *IO* = inferior oblique; *IR* = inferior rectus; *SO* = superior oblique.)

detail. Figure 12 illustrates the technique. The patient's eyes follow the examiner's finger as it is moved into each of the six positions indicated in the diagram. In each of these positions, one pair of extraocular muscles (one muscle from each eye) is in a position of maximum activity; the other muscles are acting least. In effect, each position emphasizes the function of one muscle pair so that abnormalities are revealed. Each pair of corresponding muscles constitutes a *yoke*, and one should think in terms of these six yokes when evaluating extraocular muscle function. Weakness of at least a moderate degree is usually evident without special tests.

Diplopia due to organic disease of the oculomotor system is abolished when either eye is closed. Often the patient has noticed this and comments on it during the history taking. Diplopia, or multiple images seen with one eye alone, results from an abnormality of the eye itself; sometimes the condition is psychogenic. *Diplopia is always more pronounced, i.e., the images are most widely separated, when the patient is looking toward the field of action of the weak muscle.* If the two images are side by side, either a medial or lateral rectus muscle is affected; if one is above the other, the involved muscle is one of the obliques or a superior or inferior rectus. Figure 13 shows that as the patient looks to the left, the images are widely separated, but as he looks straight ahead or to the right, he sees only one image.

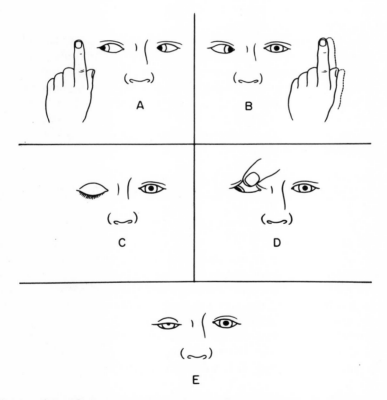

FIG. 13. (A, B) Left lateral rectus paralysis. Note double image when patient gazes in direction of action of this muscle. (C, D) Right oculomotor nerve lesion. Note complete ptosis, dilated pupil, eye abducted and depressed. (E) Right Horner's syndrome. There is slight ptosis and a constricted pupil on the right.

When the patient complains of diplopia, but weakness of the extraocular muscles is too mild to detect by ordinary examination, the
retinal images can be studied separately by covering one eye with
transparent colored material, such as red cellophane or glass, so that
the image of a light will appear red to one eye and white to the other
(the "red glass" test). The patient then moves his eyes into the six
cardinal positions, and the point at which the images are most widely
separated will then establish the involved muscle yoke. The image
from the eye with the weak muscle will be projected peripheral to
the image from the normal eye. For example, if a lateral rectus muscle
is weak, the image from that eye will be projected more laterally than
the image in the normal eye; on the other hand, if a medial rectus
muscle is weak, the image from that eye will be projected more
medially (toward the midline).

As the eyes turn to the six cardinal positions, look carefully for
nystagmus (see p. 39), rhythmic repetitive jerking movements of
the two eyes. Nystagmus is described according to the direction of
the quick component; for example, "horizontal nystagmus on right
lateral gaze, quick component to the right." A few beats of nystagmus
are normal when the patient turns his eyes into any extreme position,
but abnormal when the deviation is moderate or when the eyes are
gazing straight ahead.

Clinicoanatomic Correlations

The nuclei of the oculomotor nerves are in the midbrain, their axons
passing ventrally to emerge from the midbrain in the interpeduncular
fossa (Fig. 14). As they course through the midbrain, they pass
through the red nucleus and a portion of the cerebral peduncle. Consequently, a lesion in this region may cause, in addition to disturbances of the oculomotor nerve, abnormal movements due to involvement of the red nucleus, and possibly sensory and motor abnormalities
due to involvement of the cerebral peduncle, which carries motor and
sensory fibers to the arms and legs.

The nerve then enters the cavernous sinus (Fig. 15), where it lies
in the lateral wall near the internal carotid artery, and eventually
leaves the skull through the *superior orbital fissure* and passes into
the orbit.

The nuclei of the trochlear nerves are also in the midbrain, caudal
to the nuclei of the oculomotor nerves. Fibers turn dorsally and cross
the midline; they emerge from the dorsal surface of the midbrain and
then swing downward around the cerebral peduncle, pass into the
cavernous sinus and subsequently into the superior orbital fissure and
the orbit to innervate the superior oblique muscles.

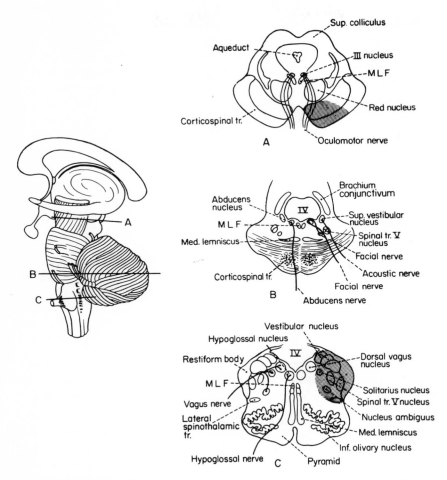

FIG. 14. Lateral view of brainstem. Lines *A, B,* and *C* indicate levels of cross sections A, B, and C. (A) Cross section of midbrain at level of superior colliculus. Shaded area indicates site of lesion producing Weber's syndrome (p. 105). (B) Cross section of pons at level of nucleus of facial nerve. (C) Cross section of medulla at level of midolive. Shaded area indicates portion damaged in Wallenberg's syndrome (p. 107). (*MLF* = medial longitudinal fasciculus.)

The nuclei of the abducens nerves lie beneath the floor of the fourth ventricle in the lower pons (see Fig. 14). Fibers are uncrossed and pass ventrally through the pons, emerging near the midline, then pass over the petrous portion of the temporal bone into the cavernous sinus and through the superior orbital fissure into the orbit to innervate the lateral rectus muscles. The nuclei of the abducens nerves are very close

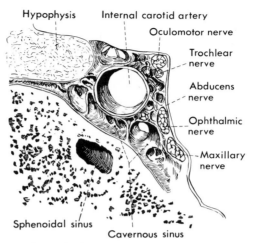

FIG. 15.   Cross section of the left cavernous sinus, showing location of internal carotid artery; oculomotor, trochlear, and abducens nerves; and the ophthalmic and maxillary branches of the trigeminal nerve.

to fibers from the facial nerve nucleus supplying the muscles of facial expression; therefore, lesions in this region usually cause both abducens and facial nerve dysfunction on the side of the lesion. Also, within the pons the fibers of the abducens nerves are in close relationship to the corticospinal tract, which carries impulses for voluntary action of the arm and leg on the opposite side. Therefore, a combination of homolateral weakness of the lateral rectus muscle with contralateral hemiplegia would suggest pontine localization. The abducens nerve has a long course after it leaves the brainstem, and because of this and its close relation to the temporal bone, it may be stretched as a result of increased intracranial pressure. In such cases, weakness of the lateral rectus muscle on one or both sides is not a localizing sign but simply a reflection of increased intracranial pressure.

In the cavernous sinus, all these nerves lie close to the internal carotid artery, and lesions of this vessel, usually aneurysms, may affect any or all of these nerves as well as the upper two divisions of the trigeminal (fifth cranial) nerve (see Fig. 15).

Individual Nerve Lesions

The oculomotor nerve supplies the levator of the upper lid (levator palpebrae superioris); the superior, inferior, and medial rectus muscles; the inferior oblique muscle; and the sphincter of the pupil. Therefore, with a complete oculomotor nerve lesion the eye cannot gaze in any of the directions in which these muscles normally turn the eye (see Fig. 13). The eyeball is usually turned downward and slightly outward because of the unopposed action of the superior oblique and lateral rectus muscles. The upper lid completely covers the eye. The pupil is dilated and does not react to light. The commonest causes of oculomotor nerve defects are diabetes mellitus and aneurysms of the internal carotid or posterior communicating arteries. With diabetes, however, the pupil is usually spared.

The trochlear nerve supplies the superior oblique muscle; isolated lesions of this nerve are uncommon. A slight impairment of downward gaze is usually present, and the patient may hold his head tilted toward the opposite side to compensate for the lack of this muscle's normal rotatory action about the anteroposterior axis of the eyeball.

The abducens nerve supplies the lateral rectus muscle. Lesions of this nerve result in inability to turn the involved eye laterally (abduct) (see Fig. 13). When the patient gazes straight ahead, the affected eye may deviate medially because the medial rectus muscle is unopposed. The patient's head may be turned slightly toward the side of the paralyzed muscle as a compensating mechanism. When this muscle is impaired, it is difficult to evaluate the superior and inferior rectus muscles, since their purest action occurs only when the eyeball is fully abducted.

Conjugate Gaze Paresis

In addition to the strabismus resulting from weakness of an individual extraocular muscle, certain lesions result in weakness of *conjugate* gaze; that is, impairment of the gaze of the two eyes together in a given direction. Impairment of conjugate gaze usually results from disease of the central nervous system rather than of the peripheral nerves or muscles. There is no double vision because the eyes remain aligned and parallel. Lesions destroying the frontal cerebral cortex anterior to the motor strip (area 8) will result in inability to gaze toward the opposite side and frequently cause deviation of the patient's eyes toward the side of the frontal cortex lesion. On the other hand, irritation of this area, as from a convulsive seizure or an infection, may produce the opposite effect—that is, forced deviation toward the opposite side. Destruction of certain lower pontine regions adjacent to the abducens nerve nucleus on one side will result in inability to gaze toward the side of the lesion and a tendency for persistent conjugate deviation toward the opposite side. With frontal lobe lesions, paresis of conjugate gaze is not usually persistent, since alternate pathways take over to alleviate the defect, but brainstem lesions often lead to permanent disability with respect to this function.

Another disturbance of conjugate gaze results from a lesion, usually a pinealoma, in the region of the *pineal gland* dorsal to the superior colliculi. Pressure on the colliculi results in inability to gaze upward (and, as pressure increases, downward as well). This is one of the most important localizing signs of upper midbrain lesions and is termed *Parinaud's syndrome*. In addition to the inability to look up and down, the pupils may be dilated. Increased intracranial pressure due to obstruction of the aqueduct of Sylvius and complete involvement of the oculomotor nerves may result as the lesion expands.

Muscle Diseases

Myasthenia gravis, a disease of the neuromuscular junction, is another important cause of weakness of the extraocular muscles. In most cases the weakness involves more than one muscle and cannot be fitted into the pattern of a discrete oculomotor, trochlear, or abducens nerve lesion. Ptosis is common, but the pupil is not affected. *Hyperthyroidism* may also lead to disorders of the extraocular muscles and to protrusion of the eyeball (proptosis or exophthalmos). Certain hereditary *muscular dystrophies* may result in ptosis and in weakness of the extraocular muscles.

Horner's Syndrome

Sympathetic nerve fibers which cause dilatation of the pupil begin in the hypothalamus, pass down the brainstem into the cervical and upper thoracic region of the spinal cord, then leave the cord, pass into the sympathetic chain, and course upward to form a network around the internal carotid artery, thereby gaining access into the skull. Within the skull they pass to the pupillodilator muscles in the iris and to the smooth muscles of the eyelids. Lesions of this pathway in the brainstem, spinal cord, or sympathetic chain cause Horner's syndrome (see Fig. 13), which consists of mild ptosis resulting from involvement of the smooth muscle of the upper lid, constriction of the pupil on the same side, and absence of sweating on the same side of the face. Horner's syndrome is an important localizing sign. It most commonly results from vascular lesions in the brainstem, cervical spinal cord injuries and tumors, and tumors and trauma affecting the sympathetic fibers in the neck. The mild ptosis is abolished as the patient gazes upward, because the levator of the upper eyelid is intact. Ptosis from weakness of the levator palpebrae superioris is not likely to lessen on upward gaze.

Pupillary Abnormalities

The *Argyll-Robertson pupil* is one of the classic neurologic pupillary abnormalities. In its complete form, the pupils are very small, and irregular rather than round; they do not react to light but do react normally to accommodation. The sign may appear in incomplete forms, and it sometimes occurs in combination with other extraocular muscle abnormalities such as ptosis. Usually both pupils are involved. The most common cause is tabes dorsalis, a form of syphilis of the central nervous system, but the abnormality has been reported in association with several other diseases.

Adie's syndrome is another pupillary abnormality which occasionally develops, usually in young women. A curious but benign disorder of unknown cause, usually affecting one eye, the syndrome consists of enlargement of the pupil and delayed and very slow reaction to light (tonic response). The pupil also reacts slowly to accommodation, but on sustained accommodation the pupil may become smaller than the normal one. For unknown reasons, the muscle stretch reflexes are often absent in this syndrome. The disorder usually begins abruptly. The patient may note slight blurring of vision because of uneven accommodation on near vision between the two eyes, but adaptation occurs and the condition is then usually asymptomatic. Its importance lies in the differential diagnosis of lesions which affect the oculomotor nerve, such as aneurysm and neurosyphilis, which also cause pupillary dilatation.

Nystagmus

Nystagmus may be an important sign of abnormality in the nervous system or the inner ear, but it is not of major localizing value except in relation to disturbances in brainstem or vestibulocerebellar connections. Any disturbance of the intricate connections between the vestibular system and the extraocular muscle nuclei may result in nystagmus. Perhaps the most common cause is the use of drugs such as barbiturates and tranquilizers. Lesions of one cerebellar hemisphere or one side of the brainstem, for example, a cerebellopontine angle tumor, may cause coarse nystagmus when the patient gazes toward the side of the lesion and finer nystagmus when he gazes toward the opposite side. Inflammation or damage to the labyrinth often causes nystagmus in association with severe vertigo and nausea. Multiple sclerosis, because of patchy involvement of many of the brainstem connections, is a common cause of nystagmus. Diseases which caused markedly reduced vision from birth may result in a pendular, rhythmic nystagmus without a quick or slow component as a consequence of defective fixation.

A specific variety of nystagmus is seen in the *medial longitudinal fasciculus syndrome*, also called *internuclear ophthalmoplegia*. The medial longitudinal fasciculus is a complex pathway which integrates the nuclei of the nerves supplying the extraocular muscles as well as impulses from the vestibular system and other portions of the nervous system related to the orientation of the body in space and the coordination between head, eye, and trunk musculature (Fig. 16). If a lesion occurs on one side in this pathway it will produce impaired adduction of the eyeball on that side and nystagmus in the opposite eye. This syndrome is usually bilateral. It is an important localizing sign because it places a lesion between the abducens and oculomotor

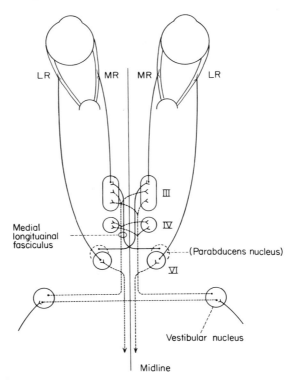

FIG. 16. Internuclear and vestibular components of the medial longitudinal fasciculus. The left MLF is circled. Lesion at this point produces paresis of adduction of the left eye and nystagmus in right eye on gaze to the right.

nerve nuclei in the brainstem. By far the most common cause is multiple sclerosis.

THE TRIGEMINAL NERVE (CRANIAL NERVE V)

The trigeminal nerve mediates general sensation, including perception of pain, temperature, and touch, for the intracranial cavity above the tentorium, the entire face and scalp to the vertex, the paranasal sinuses, and the nasal and oral cavities. It carries the afferent arc of the corneal reflex and both the afferent and efferent arcs of the jaw reflex. It also supplies motor innervation to all the muscles of mastication.

Technique of Examination

Before evaluating the sensory functions of the trigeminal nerve, visualize the distribution of its three major divisions: ophthalmic, maxillary, and mandibular (Fig. 17). Then, with the patient's eyes shut, test an area within the distribution of each of these primary divisions on each side of the face with pin and with cotton, always comparing one side with the other. Loss of perception of nasal tickle, tested by lightly brushing the base of each nostril with a wisp of cotton, may give early evidence of abnormality of the maxillary division. Temperature perception need not be evaluated unless there is an equivocal test of pain perception, since these sensory impulses travel in the same tracts. If an area of sensory loss is found, its margins should be deter-

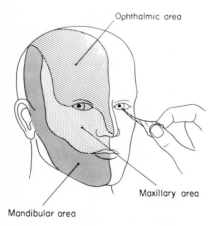

Ophthalmic area

Maxillary area

Mandibular area

FIG. 17. Distribution of trigeminal nerve innervation to the face, and technique of eliciting corneal reflex. Note sparing of angle of the jaw.

mined by proceeding outward in various directions from the area of loss until an area of normal sensation is found. The area of abnormality should be sketched on the patient's record.

An area of sensory loss due to organic disease of the trigeminal nerve or its central connections should be about the same from one examination to the next, and its outline should conform to an area innervated by this nerve. In particular, the angle of the jaw should not be involved; also, the area that is involved should not stop at the hairline, as it may in nonorganic sensory loss.

The corneal reflex should be tested in each eye. The patient's eyes should be turned away in order to avoid involuntary blinking as the stimulus approaches. A small wisp of cotton with a fine point is brought in from one side to touch the cornea (*not* the conjunctiva or eyelashes), as in Figure 17. The normal response is a bilateral blink, since the afferent arc of this reflex connects with both facial nerve nuclei. The facial nerves innervate the orbicularis oculi muscles, which act to close the eyes.

To test the jaw reflex, the mouth should be partially open and the muscles of mastication relaxed. The examiner's thumb is placed on the midline of the mandible below the lower lip and tapped sharply with a reflex hammer. Normally the reflex often cannot be elicited; when present, it consists of brisk elevation of the mandible. The jaw reflex is physiologically similar to the muscle-stretch reflexes obtained elsewhere and has the same clinical significance (see p. 79).

To evaluate the muscles of mastication, first observe and feel the region of the masseter and temporalis muscles on each side to detect unilateral and bilateral atrophy. During this procedure, have the patient clench his teeth. Then ask him to open his mouth; if the jaw muscles on one side are weak, the mandible will deviate toward the affected side and he will be unable to move his jaw toward the opposite side. The deviation results from the unbalanced rotatory action of the opposite muscles.

When the examination is finished, the extent of the area of sensory and motor deficits should be determined and a judgment made as to whether it conforms to a division of a nerve, the entire peripheral trigeminal distribution, or to central sensory pathways.

Clinicoanatomic Correlations

The nuclei of the sensory neurons of the trigeminal nerve are in the gasserian ganglion, a large collection of cell bodies lying a short distance anterior to the pons and posterior to the cavernous sinus on either side. The nuclei of the motor portion of the nerve are in the midpons. Several features of the connections within the brainstem are of clinical importance. Fibers carrying pain and temperature sensation enter the brainstem from the gasserian ganglion and pass into the spinal tract of the trigeminal nerve, which begins in the middle of the pons and descends through the pons and medulla into the upper cervical portion of the spinal cord. Synapses occur throughout this tract with neurons of the spinal nucleus of the trigeminal nerve, which carry these sensations upward to higher brain centers (secondary ascending tracts of the trigeminal nerve). Fibers carrying touch sensation terminate in the chief sensory nucleus of the trigeminal nerve, a collection of cell bodies in the midpons near the point of entrance of the nerve. Therefore, lesions in the brainstem below this nucleus may cause loss of pain and temperature sensation on that side of the face without impairing touch, in contrast to lesions peripheral to the brainstem, in which all sensory modalities may be affected.

Descending fibers from the cerebral cortex controlling voluntary movement of the mandible are both crossed and uncrossed; therefore, a lesion of this pathway (corticobulbar tract) on one side does not cause significant weakness of the jaw muscles. Weakness of these muscles almost always results from lesions of the motor nucleus or peripheral nerve, or from primary muscle diseases.

The intracranial course of the trigeminal nerve proximal to the gasserian ganglion is short, but tumors in the posterior fossa may affect this portion, usually resulting in sensory loss in all divisions of the nerve. Lesions distal to the gasserian ganglion produce deficits only in the area supplied by the affected division.

Because the ophthalmic division passes through the cavernous sinus and the superior orbital fissure, lesions of these structures result in loss of sensation in this division and in abnormalities of the extraocular muscles, since the oculomotor, trochlear, and abducens nerves also pass through the same areas (see Fig. 15). The maxillary division passes through the *foramen rotundum* on the floor of the middle cranial fossa and is then distributed to the palate, the maxillary sinus, the maxillary teeth, and the skin of the upper lip and cheek. The mandibular division passes through the *foramen ovale* and then to the mandible, the mandibular teeth, and the skin of the mandibular region. Numbness of the chin, an uncommon but important organic complaint, may be the first sign of a tumor involving the mandibular division in the region of the foramen ovale.

Lesions of the ascending tracts of the trigeminal nerve or higher pathways mediating facial sensation may produce sensory loss in the opposite side of the face. The sensory loss usually involves the entire half of the head rather than the trigeminal distribution. Sensory loss resulting from lesions of the central pathways is almost always accompanied by similar defects on the body.

Diseases Affecting the Trigeminal Nerve

Tumors located in the posterior fossa are an important cause of trigeminal nerve dysfunction. Loss of corneal reflex and facial sensation may be the first signs of such a tumor, appearing at a time when it may be removed most easily. The tumor that most commonly affects the trigeminal nerve is the acoustic neuroma, which arises in the cerebellopontine angle.

With tumors in the region of the foramina of exit of the three trigeminal divisions, loss of sensation over the related areas may occur early in the course of the disease. Tumors of the gasserian ganglion itself often cause pain in the face as well as loss of sensation.

Trigeminal neuralgia (tic douloureux), which occurs usually in persons over 50, is characterized by brief but excruciating pains, often occurring in rapid succession, in one or more divisions of the nerve, usually either maxillary or mandibular. The pain is sometimes triggered by a very mild stimulus, such as shaving or simply touching the face, and may occur repetitively for a few minutes or for hours. Examination of trigeminal nerve function discloses no abnormality even during the severe pain. It is a distinctive syndrome, and although remission may occur spontaneously, the condition causes great disability until medical or surgical treatment is given.

Herpes zoster (shingles) is caused by a virus infection of any of the sensory ganglia of the body, including the gasserian ganglion of the trigeminal nerve. The disease is manifested by a papulovesicular rash which usually involves the ophthalmic division, occasionally damaging the cornea. The rash heals but may leave a chronic painful condition called postherpetic neuralgia. Sensation may be lost over the affected area.

Disorders Affecting the Jaw Musculature

Myasthenia gravis, a disease causing weakness and fatigability of muscles, can affect the muscles of mastication to a severe degree, so that the patient is restricted to a semisolid or liquid diet. In milder cases, chewing is possible for a few moments, but the muscles soon fatigue and the meal cannot be completed.

Amyotrophic lateral sclerosis, a degenerative disease affecting motor nerve cells, is another disorder sometimes involving the jaw muscles. If it attacks the motor nucleus of the trigeminal nerve, weakness and wasting of the jaw muscles result, with consequent inability to close the mouth and to chew.

Pseudobulbar palsy, a condition resulting from bilateral destruction of the corticobulbar pathways leading to the motor nuclei of certain cranial nerves, causes a syndrome which superficially resembles a disease of these nuclei themselves. Muscles of the jaw, the face, the palate, the pharynx, and the tongue may be weak; in this condition, the jaw reflex is hyperactive because of damage to the pathways which normally inhibit this reflex. There is also emotional lability—spontaneous crying and laughing—because of damage to pathways which normally inhibit and modulate these reactions. The muscle weakness is not accompanied by wasting, because the lesion does not affect the cell bodies or axons of the lower motor neurons.

Tetanus (lockjaw) may cause severe spasm (trismus) of the muscles of mastication.

THE FACIAL NERVE (CRANIAL NERVE VII)

The facial nerve innervates all the muscles of facial expression—smiling, whistling, wrinkling the nose, closing the eyes, frowning, grimacing, and the many variations of these functions. The nerve also carries fibers mediating taste perception from the anterior portion of the tongue and innervating certain salivary glands and the lacrimal glands. The functions of the facial nerve are easily evaluated, and information of considerable significance is often obtained, since this nerve is commonly involved in diseases of the nervous system.

Technique of Examination

The most important part of the facial nerve examination is the evaluation of the muscles of facial expression. Weakness can be noted by observing the patient's face. Mild asymmetry of the face may be normal, but drooping of one side of the mouth, flattening of the nasolabial fold, and sagging of the lower eyelid suggest weakness of the facial muscles. As the patient talks, the weak side of the face does not move normally. Occasionally, the face is pulled toward the normal side. In some cases blinking is impaired; the eye may not completely close on the affected side.

To test the strength of the facial muscles, begin by asking the patient to lift his eyebrows, then to lower them. Mild weakness of the frontalis muscle is easily detected when the eyebrows do not rise symmetrically. The usual forehead wrinkles are less prominent on the weak side; if weakness is severe the difference may be striking. Next, test the orbicularis oculi muscles by asking the patient to close his eyes tightly, noting unilateral or bilateral loss of normal power of this movement. If the examiner attempts to pull the eyes open while the patient holds them shut tightly, mild weakness may be detected. If weakness is severe, the eye does not close completely. In such instances, as the patient attempts to close his eyes the normal upward rolling of the eyeball may be visible (*Bell's phenomenon*), which is not the case when strength is normal because the eyes are concealed.

The patient is next asked to smile or to show his teeth. Weakness of retraction of the mouth and of the usual smiling expression is easily seen. Asymmetry of retraction may be noted with unilateral weakness. The patient may be asked to whistle, another movement requiring normal strength of the muscles around the mouth.

During vigorous retraction of the mouth, contraction of the thin sheetlike muscle covering the anterior surface of the neck may be seen—the platysma. This paired muscle is also innervated by the facial nerve. Weakness of the platysma on one side is occasionally an early sign of dysfunction of the nerve.

When evaluating strength of the facial musculature, particular attention should be paid to the distribution of the weakness. Weakness of all of the muscles on one side of the face implies a lesion in *the facial nerve or its nucleus* (lower motor neuron). Weakness of the muscles about the mouth on one side with normal function of the upper muscles, particularly the frontalis, suggests that the lesion lies in the pathway from the opposite cerebral cortex to the nucleus of the facial nerve (the upper motor neuron).

The sense of taste should be evaluated when evidence of a lesion of the facial nerve is noted, when a lesion of the brainstem is suspected, and whenever the patient complains of an abnormality of taste. To test this function, use an applicator stick previously dipped in a salty, sweet, sour, or bitter solution. Place the applicator on one side of the tongue and ask the patient to indicate by moving his hand whether he recognizes or is aware of a taste. He should rinse his mouth with water after each test. Repeat on the other side of the tongue.

Special procedures are available to test the functions of the lacrimal and salivary glands. These functions are occasionally impaired when there are lesions of the facial nerve near its exit from the pons.

Clinicoanatomic Correlations

The motor nucleus of the facial nerve lies in the lateral portion of the lower pons. Its axons loop around the nucleus of the abducens nerve and then leave the pons near its junction with the medulla. This close relationship between the two nerves is significant because a lesion within the brainstem involving one is apt to involve the other; therefore, a combination of abducens and facial nerve dysfunction indicates a lesion in the lower portion of the pons. At their point of exit from the pons, the motor fibers are accompanied by incoming sensory fibers conveying taste and by parasympathetic fibers that innervate the lacrimal and salivary glands.

The facial nerve enters the temporal bone through the internal auditory meatus and during its course through this bone is subject to trauma from fractures of the base of the skull. It also lies in close relationship to the middle ear and therefore may be affected by diseases or surgical procedures in that area. The fibers carrying taste sensation and the fibers innervating the lacrimal and salivary glands leave the nerve as it passes through the temporal bone, so that any injury or other lesion of the nerve proximal to this point may affect taste and the secretion of these glands. Therefore, accurate testing of taste and of lacrimal secretion may aid in localizing a lesion of this nerve.

The facial nerve leaves the skull through the stylomastoid foramen and immediately passes into the substance of the parotid gland; therefore, diseases of this gland may affect some of the peripheral branches of the facial nerve. Lesions along the course of the facial nerve from its origin to the stylomastoid foramen produce weakness of all the muscles on the affected side of the face. Lesions distal to this point may cause localized weakness, depending on the specific peripheral branches involved. These are rare except in facial trauma.

Nerve impulses from the cerebral cortex which control voluntary movements of the face descend in a pathway called the corticobulbar tract. Some of these fibers cross over to terminate at the opposite facial nucleus, while others stay on the same side and terminate on the ipsilateral facial nucleus. That portion of each facial nerve nucleus which receives fibers from both the contralateral and ipsilateral cerebral cortex contains neurons which innervate the upper portion of the facial musculature, particularly the frontalis and much of the orbicularis oculi. That portion of each facial nerve nucleus receiving fibers from only the opposite cerebral cortex innervates the lower portion of the facial musculature, i.e., the perioral muscles. Therefore, a lesion of one corticobulbar tract in its course from the cerebral cortex to the pons will cause weakness of the lower facial muscles on the opposite side but will spare the muscles of the forehead.

Weakness of the face resulting from a lesion of the corticobulbar tract (upper motor neuron) is termed *central facial weakness;* weakness of the face resulting from a lesion of the facial nerve nucleus or its peripheral fibers (lower motor neuron) is called *peripheral facial weakness*. To repeat, differentiation between the two is based on the distribution of weakness of the face: A lower motor neuron lesion causes weakness of the entire half of the face on the side of the lesion, whereas an upper motor neuron lesion results in weakness only of the lower half of the face on the opposite side. This is an extremely important distinction, and the differentiation should be kept clearly in mind.

An interesting feature of the upper motor neuron variety of facial weakness is that involuntary contractions of the facial muscles, as in spontaneous smiling or laughing, may show normal strength even though the voluntary or deliberate use of the muscles is weak. Preservation of alternate pathways from other brain centers, such as the hypothalamus, accounts for the intact emotional response. It is also noteworthy that weakness from upper motor neuron lesions is rarely as severe as in lower motor neuron disorders.

The most common cause of central facial paresis is an infarct in the opposite cerebral hemisphere, but it also develops from any lesion, such as a tumor or abscess, interrupting the corticobulbar pathway from the cerebral cortex to the pons. Pseudobulbar palsy (see p. 45) results from bilateral corticobulbar tract lesions causing bilateral facial weakness as well as weakness of other cranial nerve musculature.

Peripheral facial palsy, when it has an acute onset and no evident cause, is termed *Bell's palsy*. It has been suggested that Bell's palsy is caused by swelling of the facial nerve within the temporal bone as the result of a virus infection or an allergic response. Tumors of the brainstem and in the cerebellopontine angle, fracture of the temporal bone, infection of the mastoid and middle ear, and parotid gland tumors are other disorders that may result in peripheral facial weakness. Bilateral peripheral facial weakness often develops in myasthenia gravis and in the Guillain-Barré syndrome, an acute disease of the peripheral nervous system producing widespread paralysis.

THE ACOUSTIC NERVE (CRANIAL NERVE VIII)

The acoustic nerve has two divisions—the *cochlear*, which mediates hearing; and the *vestibular*, which transmits impulses from the labyrinths of the inner ears, influencing balance, maintenance of body position, and orientation in space. Lesions in the cochlear division cause hearing loss, tinnitus (noises, usually ringing in the ear), or both. Loss of hearing in both ears usually becomes apparent to the patient early in its development; however, loss that is limited to one ear may become severe before the patient is aware of it.

Acute dysfunction of the vestibular system is apparent to the patient, who experiences vertigo, nausea, and vomiting. If the lesion develops insidiously, the patient may be unaware of a completely non-functioning labyrinth. Patients with hearing loss due to involvement of the cochlear nerve (neurogenic hearing loss) often will speak too loudly or too softly, because of inadequate feedback of the sound. This is not as common with impaired transmission of sound through the external or middle ear (conductive hearing loss), since conduction of the sound through the bones of the skull may furnish some clues as to the proper modulation of the voice. Patients with either type of hearing loss often turn their normal ear toward the speaker.

Technique of Examination

The best single screening test for hearing loss is the perception of a whisper. Cover one of the patient's ears with your hand and softly whisper a few words near the opposite ear. If the patient is easily able to understand a very soft whisper, he is not likely to have significant hearing loss in that ear. Repeat the test in the other ear. A ticking watch is sometimes recommended; however, it gives only a high tone, and as people grow older they tend to lose the ability to perceive such tones (presbycusis).

If hearing loss is detected, it is important to determine whether it results from a disease interfering with the transmission of sound from the environment to the cochlea and inner ear (conductive loss), or from a disease of the cochlea or the cochlear nerve (neurogenic loss). The *Rinné test* aids in differentiating these two varieties: A vibrating tuning fork is placed on the mastoid process and the patient indicates the point at which he no longer hears the sound. The fork is then quickly held in the air next to the patient's ear. If the patient again hears the sound, this means that the conduction mechanisms through the middle ear are intact and that the deficit lies in the inner ear or cochlear nerve. (Air conduction is better than bone conduction in normal hearing as well as in neurogenic loss.) If, on the other hand, the perception of the sound is better when the tuning fork is held on the bone, a conduction defect is implied, usually resulting from an abnormality in the middle or external ear.

The *Weber test* is also of help in differentiating between conductive and neurogenic loss. If a vibrating tuning fork is placed on the vertex of the head, the sound is normally perceived equally in both ears, or as coming from "all over the head." When conductive hearing loss is present, the sound is perceived better in the affected ear; when neurogenic loss is present, the sound will be perceived in the opposite, or normal, ear.

In addition to these simple tests, patients with hearing loss should have complete audiometric examinations to aid in determining the type of hearing loss. Other specialized tests are available for determining the site of a lesion causing hearing loss.

THE VESTIBULAR DIVISION. Specific tests of the vestibular division and its connections are not ordinarily performed unless the history or physical examination suggests disease of this system. The most important points in the patient's history include dizziness of a spinning or whirling variety (*vertigo*), which is often associated with nausea and vomiting, and unsteadiness (*ataxia*). In some cases there may be tinnitus and deafness due to associated cochlear disease.

The cold caloric test is the standard screening method for evaluating vestibular function. It is performed with the patient supine with his head elevated 30 degrees, thus placing the horizontal semicircular canal in a vertical position. First, inspect the external auditory canal and eardrum with an otoscope to make sure there is no infection or perforation of the eardrum which might be aggravated by the procedure. Then introduce 5 ml. of ice water into the canal, using an ordinary syringe and a soft-tipped rubber catheter. *Normally* this stimulus produces nystagmus, a rhythmic conjugate jerking of both eyes, with the quick component toward the opposite side of the head. It may also produce vertigo, nausea, and vomiting. If the response is decreased or absent, the vestibular system on that side is impaired. The test is performed in both ears. More elaborate tests are available to clarify disturbances in vestibular function which are not adequately defined by the cold caloric test.

Clinicoanatomic Correlations

Within the brainstem, the connections of the cochlear division are complex, including both crossed and uncrossed ascending pathways to the cerebral cortex. Therefore, lesions within the central nervous system above the level of the cochlear nuclei on one side do not produce significant hearing loss unless they are bilateral. Lesions in the cochlear nuclei on one side, however, may produce severe hearing loss. Lesions of one cerebral hemisphere, even in an area concerned with auditory perception, do not produce deafness. Since the primary auditory receptive area lies in the temporal lobe and is adjacent to the numerous complex auditory association areas, temporal lobe lesions not infrequently result in hallucinations of music, voices, or other sounds. These phenomena are among those noted in convulsive seizures resulting from tumor, trauma, or other lesions in the temporal lobe.

The vestibular system also has very complex connections within the brainstem. The vestibular nuclei are large and often are affected by brainstem diseases. Among their important connections is the intimate relationship with the *medial longitudinal fasciculus,* which connects the nuclei of the oculomotor, trochlear, and abducens nerves which innervate the extraocular muscles (see Fig. 16). Abnormal input from the vestibular system into this fiber tract can produce nystagmus. The vestibular system also has connections with nuclei in the brainstem which send nerve impulses to the abdominal and thoracic visceral organs; these connections account for the gastrointestinal, respiratory, and cardiovascular symptoms in acute diseases involving the vestibular system, such as *Meniere's syndrome,* which is associated with tinnitus, hearing loss, and episodic vertigo, nausea and vomiting.

After the acoustic nerve leaves the brainstem it is most vulnerable in the region of the internal auditory meatus, where it is near the facial nerve. A common tumor, the *acoustic neuroma* (see p. 108), arises from the nerve in this location (the cerebellopontine angle) with resulting hearing loss and tinnitus, and somewhat later, involvement of adjacent cranial nerves and the cerebellum. Fractures of the base of the skull which pass through the temporal bone frequently damage the acoustic nerve. If a basilar skull fracture damages blood vessels in the region of the middle ear, blood may accumulate behind the eardrum, or occasionally in the external auditory canal, thus providing a clue to the existence of such a fracture.

Vascular occlusions and tumors within the brainstem, as well as other tumors in the region of the lateral aspect of the pons, are also important causes of acoustic nerve dysfunction.

Motion sickness incurred during ordinary travel is caused by repetitive stimulation of the labyrinths.

GLOSSOPHARYNGEAL AND VAGUS NERVES (CRANIAL NERVES IX AND X)

These nerves are closely related both anatomically and functionally. The glossopharyngeal nerve innervates a portion of the pharyngeal musculature, conveys taste from the posterior portion of the tongue, innervates the carotid sinus and carotid body, and supplies general sensation to the tonsillar and pharyngeal mucous membranes. The vagus nerve innervates all of the thoracic and abdominal visceral organs, the larynx, the pharynx, and the palate, and it conveys numerous sensory impulses from the walls of the digestive tract, the heart, and the lungs. The visceral innervation of these nerves is very important; however, their clinical examination is directed to the motor functions of the palate, pharynx, and larynx.

Technique of Examination

The first step in the clinical evaluation is inspection of the soft palate. It should be symmetrical, and its median raphe (the pale streak in the midline) should not deviate to one side. Inspection of the uvula is less informative, because it may have been altered by tonsillectomy; also there are numerous anatomic variations ranging from complete absence of this structure to elongation and deviation to one side or the other. When the patient says "ah," the palate should rise promptly and symmetrically. Next, the posterior wall of the oropharynx is touched with a tongue depressor, to induce the *gag reflex*. This reflex includes prompt elevation of the palate, and constriction of the pharyngeal musculature and the common sensation of gagging. It

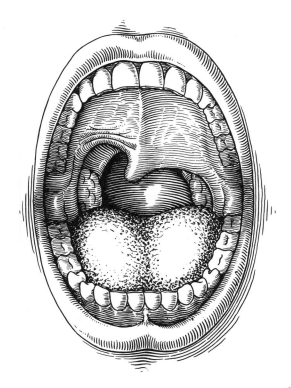

FIG. 18. Paresis of left side of palate, with contraction visible only on the right. The palate is pulled toward the normal side.

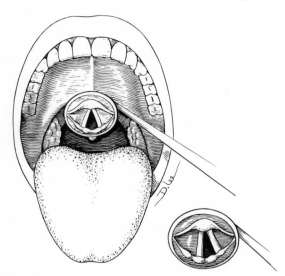

FIG. 19. Indirect laryngoscopy, showing normal appearance of vocal cords and (*inset*) paresis of right vocal cord.

shows a normal range of variability in sensitivity and is often brisk in nervous people and heavy smokers. The gag reflex should be elicited on both sides if weakness of the palate is found.

When unilateral weakness of the palate is present, the affected side will be lower and without the normal arch at its margin (Fig. 18). When the patient phonates, the palate is pulled toward the opposite side because the muscles on the normal side are unopposed.

To test the function of swallowing, have the patient swallow some water and watch for any difficulty in that action, and for regurgitation of fluid through the nose, which would indicate weakness of the soft palate and resulting inability to close off the nasopharynx.

If the patient is hoarse or complains of voice disturbance, the vocal cords should be inspected by indirect laryngoscopy with a laryngeal mirror (Fig. 19). A unilateral lesion of the vagus nerve or its nuclei in the brainstem produces paresis of the vocal cord on that side, resulting in hoarseness and abnormal phonation (see p. 13). With bilateral vagal lesions, the patient may be unable to voice any sound (aphonia), and he will also have great difficulty in swallowing. The resulting inability to handle secretions and the likelihood of aspirating food into the trachea create a life-threatening situation.

Clinicoanatomic Correlations

The routine examination of the glossopharyngeal and vagus nerves evaluates the *nucleus ambiguus*, located in the lateral portion of the medulla on both sides (see Fig. 14C).

The nucleus ambiguus receives corticobulbar innervation from both cerebral hemispheres. Consequently, a unilateral corticobulbar tract lesion produces little or no dysfunction of pharynx, palate, or larynx. Bilateral corticobulbar lesions, however, produce the syndrome of pseudobulbar palsy (see p. 45), and this may cause profound dysfunction of these structures, to a life-threatening degree in some cases because of the danger of asphyxia or aspiration pneumonia. Pseudobulbar palsy must be distinguished from *bulbar palsy*, which also causes weakness of jaw, face, palate, pharynx, larynx, and tongue. In the latter instance, however, the weakened muscles are atrophic, fasciculations are evident, and the gag reflex is absent, because the disease affects the motor nuclei themselves (lower motor neurons). Amyotrophic lateral sclerosis, poliomyelitis, and brainstem tumors are examples of diseases causing bulbar palsy.

The nucleus ambiguus is vulnerable to vascular occlusions resulting from thrombosis of the artery supplying the lateral medullary region (the posterior inferior cerebellar artery). If this artery is occluded, the lateral portion of the medulla will be deprived of its blood supply and a characteristic clinical picture results—the Wallenberg syndrome (p. 107; see also Fig. 14). Hoarseness develops abruptly, and the patient has difficulty in swallowing (dysphagia), because of damage to the nucleus ambiguus, but since this is a unilateral lesion the disability may be moderate. In addition, the arm and leg on the same side become clumsy, and there may be loss of pain and temperature perception on the same side of the face and on the opposite side of the body. Horner's syndrome (see p. 38) develops.

The glossopharyngeal, vagus, and spinal accessory nerves leave the skull through the *jugular foramen* together with the internal jugular vein; therefore, trauma or a tumor of this region may affect all these nerves. The recurrent laryngeal nerve, a branch of the vagus supplying the larynx, is vulnerable to injury during surgical operations on the thyroid because it lies adjacent to the gland.

The vagus (and usually the glossopharyngeal) nerve may be affected in many other disorders, including tumors within the posterior cranial fossa, injuries, infections, pressure from enlarged lymph nodes, and several degenerative diseases. Poliomyelitis, now rare, was once the classic example of an infection which often involved the vagus nuclei with resulting severe impairment of swallowing and laryngeal function.

Amyotrophic lateral sclerosis often affects the portion of the vagus nerve supplying the muscles of the palate, pharynx, and larynx, producing dysphagia, dysphonia, and dysarthria. Myasthenia gravis also frequently affects these muscles, resulting in nasal speech, regurgitation of fluids through the nose, dysphagia, and dysarthria.

SPINAL ACCESSORY NERVE (CRANIAL NERVE XI)

The spinal accessory nerve is a purely motor nerve supplying the sternocleidomastoid and the upper portion of the trapezius muscles. The sternocleidomastoid muscle acting on one side rotates the head so that the face is upward and to the opposite side; when both muscles act together they flex the neck. These muscles are normally powerful, but they are not essential to maintain the head erect and to rotate it. The trapezius muscle aids in lifting or shrugging the shoulder, and when both muscles act together, they brace and retract the shoulders. Perhaps the most important function of the trapezius, however, is that of rotation of the scapula when the arm is raised. This rotation turns the glenoid fossa upward, enabling the head of the humerus, in which it rests, to pivot as the arm is raised. Without the function of the trapezius the arm cannot be raised above a horizontal plane.

Technique of Examination
The nerve is evaluated by testing the strength and bulk of these two muscles on each side (Fig. 20). To test the strength of the sternocleido-

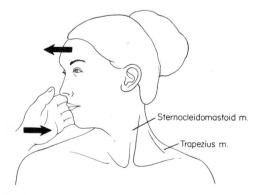

FIG. 20. Examination of the sternocleidomastoid muscle. The patient has turned her head to the right; she holds it in that position while the examiner attempts to turn it toward the front. The left sternocleidomastoid can be seen and palpated.

mastoid, the patient is asked to turn his head toward one shoulder while the examiner resists this movement. The sternocleidomastoid muscle opposite the direction of rotation is easily observed and palpated. The procedure is repeated on the other side.

The trapezius muscles are evaluated by having the patient shrug his shoulders while the examiner attempts to push them downward. Next, the patient elevates his arms to a vertical position. Weakness of the trapezius will prevent this movement. The muscles should be inspected for the presence of fasciculations and atrophy. When there is a lesion of the spinal accessory nerve, the shoulder on the affected side is considerably lower and the loss of contour is apparent.

Clinicoanatomic Correlations

Cell bodies of the spinal accessory nerve lie in the upper part of the cervical spinal cord in segments C1 through C5. This nucleus receives innervation from both cerebral hemispheres; consequently, a unilateral lesion causes little or no dysfunction.

The fibers emerge from the spinal cord on its lateral aspect between the fibers of the dorsal and ventral spinal roots. They then turn upward to form a single nerve, which passes into the posterior cranial fossa through the foramen magnum and then directly back out of the skull through the jugular foramen where it lies close to the glossopharyngeal and vagus nerves and the internal jugular vein. In lesions of this region, such as tumors, one may observe involvement of these three cranial nerves. The spinal accessory nerve then passes in the lateral aspect of the neck to the sternocleidomastoid and trapezius muscles. Trauma to the neck is the most common cause of an isolated lesion of the spinal accessory nerve.

A curious condition called *torticollis,* in which the patient's head is forcibly rotated to one side either in a constant deviation or in a jerky fashion, is caused in part by intermittent contractions of the sternocleidomastoid muscle on the opposite side. Opinions vary as to the cause of this condition, some holding that it is psychogenic, but it is most probably a disease of the basal ganglia and their connections.

THE HYPOGLOSSAL NERVE (CRANIAL NERVE XII)

The hypoglossal nerve is a purely motor nerve which innervates the tongue musculature. Normal function of the tongue is essential for normal speech and swallowing. If both sides of the tongue are weak, even if the weakness is mild, some difficulty with articulation of consonant sounds and with swallowing occurs. Severe bilateral tongue weakness causes grave difficulties with both speech and swallowing.

However, moderate or even severe weakness of only one side of the tongue may result in little or no significant clinical dysfunction.

Technique of Examination

The tongue is first examined by inspection when it is at rest in the mouth. Look for asymmetry, loss of bulk on one side or the other, deviation to one side, and fasciculations, the fine muscular twitching which may indicate a disease of the hypoglossal nerve or its nucleus. Fasciculations are often difficult to detect with the tongue protruded, since normal tremulousness may obscure these fine movements.

Next, ask the patient to protrude his tongue; it normally protrudes straight out. If the tongue turns toward one side or the other, weakness may be present on the side toward which the tongue deviates (Fig. 21). The patient is then asked to push one cheek from within with his tongue while the examiner attempts to oppose the action by pressing the patient's cheek. Normally this action can be maintained

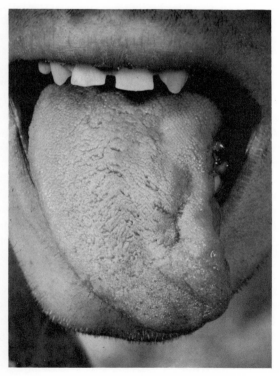

FIG. 21. Weakness of left side of tongue due to left hypoglossal nerve lesion. Note deviation toward the left on protrusion.

by the patient with surprising force. The procedure is repeated on the opposite side. Mobility and strength of the tongue may be further tested by asking the patient to elevate his tongue to touch the roof of his mouth. When dysarthria is present, coordination of the tongue should be evaluated. This is accomplished by having the patient move his tongue from side to side or in and out as rapidly as possible, or by quickly repeating "t" or "d."

Clinicoanatomic Correlations

Within the medulla, the nuclei of the hypoglossal nerves lie near the midline beneath the floor of the fourth ventricle (see Fig. 14C). These nuclei, like other nuclei of the motor components of cranial nerves V, VII, IX, X, and XI, receive innervation from the cerebral cortex of both hemispheres via the corticobulbar tracts. Remember the exception—the primarily crossed fibers of the portion of cranial nerve VII supplying the lower portion of the face. Thus, unilateral corticobulbar lesions do not produce marked weakness of the tongue, although mild weakness and deviation sometimes occur, the deviation being toward the side opposite the lesion. In pseudobulbar palsy severe tongue weakness occurs because both corticobulbar tracts are affected. Bulbar palsy (see p. 53), caused by a bilateral nuclear lesion, for example, poliomyelitis or amyotrophic lateral sclerosis, also causes severe tongue weakness, but differs from pseudobulbar palsy in that atrophy and fasciculations are present (lower motor neuron weakness).

The hypoglossal nerve may be damaged by injuries to the neck, causing unilateral lower motor neuron dysfunction with resulting unilateral weakness of the tongue, atrophy, and fasciculations. In this or in other instances of unilateral tongue weakness, the protrusion mechanism of the intact side of the tongue, when unopposed, will turn the tongue toward the weak side as it protrudes.

Occasionally, a tumor at the base of the posterior fossa of the skull near the foramen magnum may result in ipsilateral paralysis of the tongue. Another uncommon cause of unilateral tongue paralysis is a syrinx, a cavity within the medulla.

Bilateral weakness or paralysis of the tongue is more common than unilateral paralysis. Amyotrophic lateral sclerosis is one of the most common diseases causing bilateral tongue weakness. It also occurs in myasthenia gravis, a disorder of the neuromuscular junction causing fatigability and weakness of many of the muscles of the body. In this disease, however, no wasting or fasciculations accompany the weakness.

The motor system includes those parts of the nervous system directly involved with initiating, maintaining, and controlling movements of the body.

Although stimulation of the nerve to a muscle will produce contraction of that muscle, much more is involved in producing useful movement. Many delicately coordinated influences act upon the innervation of the primary muscle and also of related muscles that aid or oppose the movement.

Numerous feedback mechanisms operate to produce such a voluntary movement. Feedback impulses from the muscles travel by way of the afferent portions of the spinal nerves, entering the spinal cord to modulate the efferent outflow to the muscle. Afferent impulses ascending to the cerebellum act to suppress and modulate efferent impulses to the muscles by providing normal tonus. This allows graded contraction and relaxation of agonists, synergists, and antagonists at the various joints. The cerebellum also influences the motor portions of the cerebral cortex. The basal ganglia influence these motor circuits by means of complex connections with the thalamus, substantia nigra, reticular formation, and other areas. All of these structures contribute to the descending facilitory and inhibitory influences on the anterior horn cells (lower motor neurons).

In a system of such complexity the potential sites of malfunction are many. The symptoms and signs of specific motor lesions, however, are so characteristic that the sites may be identified by clinical examination alone, in most instances.

In the examination of the motor system, a concept of paramount importance is that concerning the distinction between the upper motor neuron and the lower motor neuron in relation to clinical signs and symptoms (Table 1).

The *upper motor neuron* is included in a system that begins in the cerebral cortex and projects downward, one part (corticobulbar tract) ending in the brainstem, the other (corticospinal tract) crossing in the lower medulla and descending in the spinal cord. The corticobulbar tract ends in the various cranial nerve nuclei. The corticospinal tract ends in the region of the anterior gray horn of the spinal cord at all levels from cervical through sacral. Those corticospinal fibers traveling through the medullary pyramids constitute the pyramidal tracts. Although certain anatomic and physiologic differences

TABLE 1.   Differentiation between upper and lower motor neuron weakness

	Upper Motor Neuron (syn.: pyramidal tract,[a] corticospinal tract, corticobulbar tract)	Lower Motor Neuron (syn.: anterior horn cell, ventral horn cell, somatic motor portions of cranial nerves, final common pathway)
Type and distribution of weakness	Lesions in brain—"pyramidal distribution," i.e., distal, esp. hand muscles, and weaker *extensors* in arm and weaker *flexors* in legs. Lesions in cord—variable, depending on location	Depends on which lower motor neurons are involved, i.e., which segments, roots, or nerves
Tone	Spasticity—greater in flexors in arms and extensors in legs	Flaccidity
Bulk	Slight atrophy of disuse only	Atrophy—may be marked
Reflexes	Accentuated; Babinski sign present	Decreased or absent; no Babinski sign
Fasciculations	No	Yes
Clonus	Frequently present	Absent

[a] Refers to fibers in the medullary pyramids.

exist, the terms *pyramidal tract* and *corticospinal tract* are often incorrectly used synonymously.

The *lower motor neuron* system includes the motor cells of the cranial nerve nuclei with their axons as well as the anterior horn cells, located in the anterior gray horn of the spinal cord, and their associated axons, the latter leaving the spinal cord in the ventral roots and forming the motor portion of the spinal nerves that innervate the body musculature.

Lesions of the upper motor neuron, in either the corticospinal or corticobulbar tract, produce a characteristic clinical picture. Weakness may be mild or severe and is accompanied by an increase in tone of the muscle, detected by movement of the joint by the examiner; this hypertonus is termed *spasticity*. An upper motor neuron lesion is also accompanied by accentuated muscle stretch reflexes in the involved muscles. A Babinski sign (see p. 84) appears with upper motor neuron lesions involving the corticospinal tract.

Lesions of the lower motor neuron (anterior horn cells or their axons) also produce a characteristic clinical picture. Weakness may be mild or severe, and in this instance it is accompanied by loss of muscle tone (hypotonus), wasting (atrophy) of the affected muscle, and fasciculations—fine, random, spontaneous twitches that are visible at the skin surface. Fasciculations are not found with upper motor neuron lesions, and atrophy occurs only with disuse of the muscle or limb and is mild. The muscle stretch reflexes are decreased or absent with lesions of the lower motor neurons.

The differences between these two types of muscle weakness must be kept clearly in mind, since the distinction is often crucial in neurologic diagnosis.

Technique of Examination

GAIT. The examiner may detect abnormalities of the motor system simply by observing the patient as he enters the examining room and while he is answering questions. Abnormalities may be revealed in clumsy or involuntary movements or a tendency to use only one arm; asymmetry of the body musculature may be noticeable. The formal examination of the motor system should begin by observing the patient walking in his natural way. Although individual gaits vary, a certain sense of rhythm and regularity are present in a normal gait.

Several important neurologic lesions result in characteristic alterations in gait. For example, the normal rhythmic swinging of the arms is reduced on the side of hemiparesis. When the lesion is located in the corticospinal tract, muscle tone is increased; therefore, the affected leg is held stiffly and tends to be circumducted as the patient walks, with the toe scraping the floor. The patient's arm may be flexed because flexor tone predominates in the upper extremities. In *parkinsonism* the posture may be one of mild flexion of most of the joints of the body. The arms do not swing and the steps are slow and short. An unsteady, staggering (ataxic) gait with the feet placed far apart (broad-based) suggests a lesion affecting the *cerebellar pathways*.

Abnormalities in strength and coordination of the walking process may be brought out by having the patient walk heel-to-toe (tandem walking). This reduces the base of support and accentuates abnormalities, particularly in coordination, which are not evident on casual walking. When the patient is standing, certain other simple tests may be performed. Having the patient walk on his heels may disclose weakness of the ankle dorsiflexors, muscles commonly involved in both upper and lower motor neuron lesions. If the patient has difficulty doing a deep knee bend or bending over to touch the floor, weakness of the hip and thigh muscles may be present.

STRENGTH. Before testing muscle strength, observe the major

muscle groups of the arms and legs and note any asymmetry between the two sides. If there is a question as to symmetry, measure the circumference of the limbs. Reduced size of one limb may indicate lower motor neuron weakness; upper motor neuron weakness produces minimal atrophy of disuse or none at all. While observing symmetry and size of the muscles, the examiner may detect fasciculations. Taken alone, the presence of fasciculations may be unimportant, since many normal people have them, particularly when tense or fatigued. (Benign fasciculations are common in medical students.) However, in the presence of weakness, wasting, and reflex abnormalities, fasciculations suggest lesions of the anterior horn cell or its axon.

Relatively few of the several hundred muscles of the body can be practically examined for strength, size, and symmetry. Musculature involved in the following movements should always be evaluated: shoulder abduction and adduction, elbow flexion and extension, wrist flexion and extension, hand grip, hip flexion and extension, knee flexion and extension, and ankle dorsiflexion. Muscles tested on one side should always be compared with the same muscles on the opposite side to afford a basis for judging unilateral weakness.

The extent of muscle strength testing depends on the patient's history and associated physical findings. For example, if the history suggests a peripheral nerve injury, then several of the muscles innervated by that nerve should be evaluated. Therefore, the examiner must accumulate localizing data as he proceeds through the examination, to aid in deciding how many muscles to evaluate.

The examiner must use both common sense and experience to determine normal strength, considering age, sex, the presence of other complicating illnesses, and extent of cooperation. Strength that is "normal" for elderly or chronically ill persons would be subnormal in a healthy college student. If the patient has pain in the muscles or joints, strength may be difficult to evaluate.

Since people vary in their ability and willingness to cooperate in vigorous muscle testing, complete objectivity is difficult to achieve. In some cases, a momentary vigorous muscle contraction is followed by sudden relaxation or "giving way" of the muscle, or the contraction is irregular and jerky rather than smooth or powerful. These features, in the absence of pain, suggest a psychologic problem.

TONE. After strength has been evaluated, the tone of each limb should be assessed. Tone refers to the resistance detected by an examiner when the patient's joint is moved through its range of motion with no active muscle contraction by the patient, and is characteristically altered in certain diseases of the nervous system. Reduction in tone is caused by diseases of the cerebellum and by diseases of the lower motor neuron. Because normal resistance is slight, hypotonus may be difficult to detect.

Increased tone is easier to evaluate. There are two general types: the spasticity resulting from upper motor neuron lesions and the rigidity associated with lesions of the basal ganglia.

Spasticity involves certain muscle groups more than others. With upper motor neuron lesions, tone in the flexor muscles of the arms is increased more than that in the extensor muscles, whereas in the leg the reverse is true. Therefore the arm is held in flexion and the leg in extension. Spasticity is often not present throughout the full excursion of a joint but only during the initial part of the movement. If a joint in such a case is rapidly extended by the examiner, initial resistance to the movement is felt, but after partial extension the examiner detects sudden lessening of resistance. This effect is known as the "clasp-knife phenomenon."

Rigidity is associated with diseases of the basal ganglia, such as parkinsonism. Generally, tone in all of the flexor muscles of the body is heightened, resulting in a flexed posture. Rigidity is found throughout the range of motion of the joint, in contrast to the clasp-knife phenomenon seen in spasticity. Other descriptive terms include "lead pipe" or "plastic" rigidity. In addition to rigidity, a superimposed rhythmic contraction of muscle groups may be felt by the examiner as he moves the joint. This is termed "cogwheel" rigidity and is commonly found in parkinsonism.

PALPATION. Patients with lower motor neuron disease or debilitation from any cause may have lax muscles. In acute inflammatory muscle diseases such as polymyositis and trichinosis, and in acute virus diseases of the neurons such as poliomyelitis, muscle pain and tenderness are common. Tenderness to palpation is also common in polyneuritis. Such muscle tenderness on palpation is of more importance in evaluation of sensory function than in the localization of motor lesions.

COORDINATION. Coordination is an integral function of the motor system. Tests of coordination are numerous, and only a few need be performed in most patients. It is important to compare coordination of one side of the body with the other.

Having the patient rapidly touch each finger with his thumb is a sensitive test of coordination. When the patient pats his hand on his thigh rapidly, slowness and decomposition of movement may be evident. This test can be made more complex by requesting alternate pronating and supinating movements of the hand when patting the thigh. Another useful test is the finger-nose test, in which the patient alternately touches the examiner's finger and his own nose rapidly. Rapid patting of the foot on the floor serves the same purpose as rapid hand patting. The heel-shin test is performed by asking the patient to place the heel of one foot on the opposite knee and slide it directly down the front of the shin to the ankle. Tandem walking, mentioned earlier, also yields information about coordination of leg and trunk muscles.

In addition to normal cerebellar function, the patient must have normal strength, tone, and sensory input in order to carry out coordinated movements, and in the presence of weakness or sensory disturbances, the tests for coordination may be impaired. The examiner must use all evidence from the history and examination to determine whether an incoordinated movement results from cerebellar disease, weakness, sensory impairment, or from a combination of factors. Mild weakness, though it may produce some difficulty in performing rapid movements, usually does not produce the decomposition, jerkiness, and irregularity characterizing diseases of the cerebellum or its connections.

INVOLUNTARY MOVEMENTS. Involuntary movements of the body and extremities may provide important diagnostic information; in some diseases of the nervous system such movements are the most important signs. They share the common characteristic of disappearing during sleep. The most common involuntary movement is *tremor*, a rhythmic alternating contraction of opposing muscle groups of an extremity or of the head, jaw, or tongue. Tremor results primarily from diseases affecting the basal ganglia, such as parkinsonism, or from diseases involving certain cerebellar connections. In basal ganglia disease, the tremor is present at rest when the patient is relaxed. Although it usually affects the fingers and hands on one or both sides, it may also affect proximal portions of the arms or legs, as well as the trunk or the head. If the patient then uses the limb, as in reaching for an object, the tremor decreases or disappears.

Lesions of cerebellar pathways result in a different type of tremor—the so-called *intention tremor*, which appears only as the patient reaches for an object, and increases as the hand nears the object. These tremors can be violent and incapacitating. A third type of tremor, most likely of basal ganglia origin, is observed when the patient holds an extremity in a fixed posture, for example, arms outstretched. This *postural tremor* is seen in hyperthyroidism, anxiety syndromes, hereditary tremor, and occasionally in parkinsonism.

Chorea is another important type of involuntary movement, most commonly present in two disorders—*Huntington's chorea* and *Sydenham's chorea*. In both, the basal ganglia and their connections are affected. Chorea consists of rapid, irregular, jerky, purposeless contractions of random muscle groups, followed by prompt relaxation. Contractions usually do not continually repeat within the same group but flit from one muscle group to another, in the face, neck, or extremities. Generally, the movements are most prominent distally. They resemble the fidgety movements observed in restless individuals, especially children; therefore, mild chorea may be misdiagnosed as "nervousness." Patients with chorea tend to hyperpronate the arms when holding them outstretched or above the head. Patients also tend to hold the hand in an unusual posture, called "dishing," in which there is hyperextension at the metacarpophalangeal joints combined with flexion at the wrist. If a person with chorea grasps the examiner's fingers, a "milking" sensation may be perceived by the examiner, because of the rapid involuntary movements of the patient's fingers. A patient with chorea may show few abnormal movements when he is sitting quietly, but if he moves around or walks, the choreic movements may be accentuated, occasionally so much so that the patient's gait becomes unsteady.

Athetosis is a movement disorder seen in patients with some forms of congenital brain damage and other uncommon neurologic diseases involving the basal ganglia. Athetotic movements are slow, writhing, twisting, and irregular, beginning in one muscle group and spreading to adjacent groups. They are usually most evident in the hands and in the face and are differentiated from chorea by their slowness and "wormlike" spread through adjacent muscle groups. They result in slow grimacing movements of the facial muscles leading to distorted expressions. The tongue may be affected and speech severely altered.

Dystonia is a movement disorder resulting from diseases of the basal ganglia in which parts of the body are held in abnormal postures for varying lengths of time. These postures result from rotatory movements—extreme pronation or supination or forced head or trunk rotation—sometimes combined with powerful flexion or extension at various joints. Dystonic movements are slow and powerful when fully developed but may be transient earlier. They may lead to fixed and severe distortions of posture of the limbs and trunk. Examples include torticollis, a forced intermittent or continuous turning of the head toward one side, and *dystonia musculorum deformans,* a rare disease with dystonic movements of many muscles of the extremities and trunk. Ingestion of certain drugs such as those of the phenothiazine group, virus infections of the brain, and some rare metabolic disorders such as Wilson's disease may result in dystonia.

Hemiballism is a rare movement disorder resulting from cerebrovascular occlusions affecting the subthalamic nucleus or its connections. The onset is abrupt. Movements are unilateral, affecting the side opposite the occlusion. The arm is most severely affected. The disorder consists of violent flinging movements at the proximal joints, sometimes so severe that the limb is injured. The patient may become exhausted. Movements are continuous in the early phase; however, their intensity usually diminishes after a few weeks.

Tic is an involuntary movement of uncertain etiology characterized by repetitive, stereotyped movements recurring in a specific group of muscles acting in their normal synergistic fashion. It is a benign disorder most commonly occurring in the muscles about the eye.

The sensory system conveys information to the central nervous system from the surface of the body and its environment (exteroception), regarding the position of the limbs and body in space (proprioception), and regarding the status of the internal organs (enteroception). Because sensory interpretation is subjective, the examiner must depend on the patient to provide reliable information.

For the sake of convenience the sensory examination is divided into the following sections, which reflect the traditional divisions of the sensory system: (1) superficial or exteroceptive, including pain, temperature, and touch sensation; (2) proprioceptive, including motion and position sense; (3) vibratory sense, which may be associated anatomically with proprioception; and (4) cortical sensory functions, which require normal input and integration of the exteroceptive and proprioceptive divisions.

In addition to abnormalities observed in these sensory functions, their distribution over the body usually conveys diagnostic information. There are specific patterns of sensory loss resulting from lesions of (1) cerebral hemisphere, (2) brainstem, (3) spinal cord, (4) posterior nerve root, (5) brachial and lumbosacral plexus, (6) single peripheral nerve, and (7) multiple distal peripheral nerves, as illustrated in Figure 22. In addition to these categories, hysterical and other psychologic difficulties can produce sensory loss of widely variable types. After presentation of the technique of examination and the related anatomy, the characteristics of these patterns will be considered.

Technique of Examination

The sensory examination may be difficult to interpret, especially if the patient is not alert and responsive. The information that it conveys is subject to wide variation, depending on the patient's ability to cooperate and the examiner's skill in adapting his techniques to the situation. The patient should be comfortable, relaxed, and unhurried; he should not be urged to respond more quickly than he can. The patient's eyes should be closed during the tests of all portions of the sensory system to avoid possibly distracting visual clues.

PAIN AND TEMPERATURE. The standard method of evaluating pain perception is to stimulate a small area of the skin with several pinpricks and ask the patient if he feels the discomfort. A person may

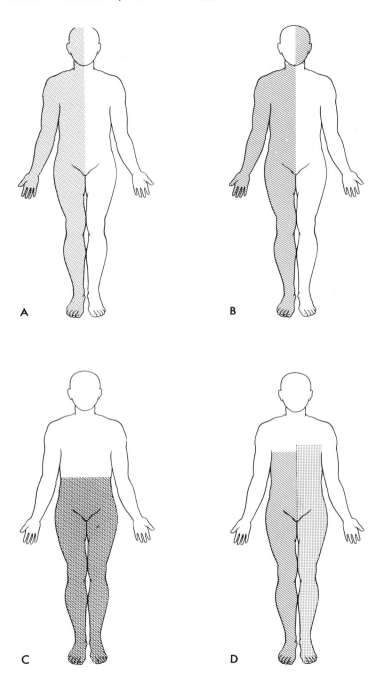

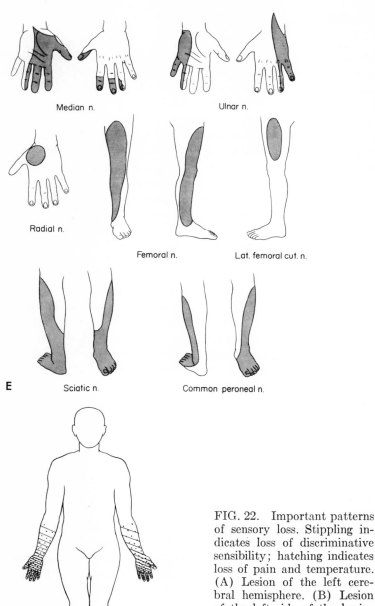

Median n.

Ulnar n.

Radial n.

Femoral n.

Lat. femoral cut. n.

E

Sciatic n.

Common peroneal n.

F

FIG. 22. Important patterns of sensory loss. Stippling indicates loss of discriminative sensibility; hatching indicates loss of pain and temperature. (A) Lesion of the left cerebral hemisphere. (B) Lesion of the left side of the brainstem. (C) Complete transverse lesion of the spinal cord. (D) Brown-Sequard syndrome, lesion on the left side of the spinal cord. (E) Lesions of important peripheral nerves. (F) Polyneuropathy.

be able to detect the touch of the pin without considering it painful; therefore, the patient must express discomfort before the response can be judged normal. If the patient's interpretation is in doubt, the sharp stimuli should be alternated with blunt, to determine whether the patient can accurately perceive a painful stimulus.

Obviously, one cannot test every square inch of the body surface; therefore, the examination must be guided by information from the patient's history, such as numbness, tingling, or "pins and needles," and by associated motor and reflex findings which suggest that sensory pathways also may be involved. The affected area must be examined in detail, so that its boundaries can be determined and conclusions drawn regarding the location of the lesion. If neither historical nor physical data indicate any sensory difficulty, a survey of the body should be made for perception of pain. This survey should include stimulation of each extremity and of the trunk, comparing one side with the other, and comparing proximal areas with distal areas on each extremity. The trunk should be surveyed on each side, and it should also be tested from inferior to superior in order to detect a level of sensory loss. When an area of sensory loss is detected, the margins are delineated by repeated pinpricks moving outward in various directions from the area of loss. The area can then be outlined with a soft wax pencil, if desired.

Deep pain, evoked by stimulating subcutaneous and deeper structures, is carried in the same central pathway as superficial pain, and lesions involving these nerves usually impair both types of pain sensation. In some instances, however, the perception of deep pain may be impaired when superficial sensation is normal, as in some cases of tabes dorsalis. Deep pain perception is tested in the legs by squeezing the Achilles tendon or the calf muscles, and in the arms by squeezing the intrinsic hand muscles.

Temperature perception travels in pathways closely related to those for pain and usually need not be tested if pain perception is normal. However, temperature perception occasionally may be altered before pain, so the test should be performed if there is reason to suspect that a lesion of the pain and temperature tracts is present. Temperature should also be tested in any situation where the patient complains of a lack of such perception, or where the patient's response to pain testing has been equivocal. Any cold or warm stimulus may be used, the standard devices being test tubes containing warm and cool water. Generally, the pattern of loss will correspond to that for pain.

TOUCH.   Ordinary touch perception is evaluated in a manner similar to the test for pain. A piece of cotton is lightly applied to the skin in various areas, and the patient is asked to respond whenever he feels the touch. The most sensitive test is to flick a single hair. In clinical practice, touch is rarely affected without loss of other sensory modalities; in fact, because multiple sensory pathways are involved, touch perception may remain intact when other sensory modalities are severely affected.

As with pain, the area of reduction in touch perception should be delineated by beginning within the area of loss and moving toward its margins in various directions. Usually, the examiner may accomplish this best by slowly dragging a wisp of cotton over the skin toward the margin of the area of sensory loss.

MOTION AND POSITION. The sense of joint motion and position, a proprioceptive modality, is tested in every extremity in the same fashion. The distal phalanx of one of the digits is grasped and slowly flexed or extended. The patient is asked to state when the examiner begins to move it. The patient is then asked to indicate whether the joint movement is upward or downward. This test is very sensitive. Check the technique on yourself or another healthy person. A minute movement of the distal phalanx of the finger (only slightly greater in the toe) is quickly detected. Initially the joint is moved through small arcs; if errors are made the arcs are increased. If position sense is severely impaired, the patient may not be able to detect movements of even the proximal joints such as the ankle or knee. Position sense is always lost distally in organic lesions; therefore, if the perception is normal for distal joints it is not necessary to test proximal joints.

The *Romberg test* evaluates sense of position of the legs and trunk. Ask the patient to stand with his feet together and his eyes open; after noting any imbalance, ask the patient to close his eyes. If the patient then sways markedly, or sidesteps to keep his balance, the test is positive and indicates an abnormality in the proprioceptive pathways. He can remain steady when he has his eyes open because the visual orientation substitutes for proprioceptive information. In contrast, patients with cerebellar disorders may sway or stagger with their eyes open as well as closed.

VIBRATION. The pathways carrying the sense of vibration are not fully delineated; they may be related to those carrying motion and position sense. A vibrating tuning fork, preferably of low amplitude (128 Hz.), is placed against a bony prominence in each of the extremities. In the legs either the internal or external malleolus may be used, and in the arms any of the finger joints are satisfactory. The patient is asked to indicate whether or not he feels the vibration. The examiner must be certain that the patient understands that the perception of vibration is required, rather than pressure or touch. The vibration should be minimal initially, with increasing strength if perception is lacking. By timing the duration of the perception, a rough quantitation may be achieved.

Young people should be able to feel a minimal vibration from the fork, but in elderly persons the sensation is usually reduced, especially in the distal portion of the legs. If the patient's judgment is in doubt, the tuning fork should occasionally be applied to the area tested without any vibration, in order to determine whether the touch of the instrument is being reported as vibration. As with motion and position sense, if the vibration is perceived at distal sites on the extremity, it is unnecessary to test proximal areas.

In some cases, the test of vibration sense may offer significant clues to the presence of nonorganic disease. For example, where there is presumed loss of sensation on one side of the body and head, the patient may indicate lack of perception of vibration on the affected side of the forehead but normal perception on the other, a situation which cannot be obtained in organic disease since the transmission of the vibration occurs immediately throughout the bony structures. The same principle applies when the test involves the mandible or the sternum. Occasionally, patients with nonorganic disorders may perceive vibration normally at the hand or wrist but not at the elbow or shoulder.

CORTICAL SENSORY PERCEPTION. The preceding sensory modalities constitute basic sensory information entering the brain, aside from visceral sensation and the special senses of vision, hearing, olfaction, and taste. The information is integrated and interpreted in the sensory (mostly parietal) cortex. Although the function is termed *cortical* perception, similar disturbances can result from lesions of the subcortical white matter of the cerebral hemispheres. Thus, the term *cortical* is not used in its strict anatomic definition of "gray" versus "white" matter, but rather to identify higher cerebral centers of integration beyond the thalamus. Specific sensory functions can easily be evaluated for information regarding the sensory cortex (see Fig. 1), but only if transmission of the primary information from the periphery is unimpaired. For example, if the primary sensory modalities are reduced because of a peripheral nerve lesion affecting the hand, lack of recognition of objects placed in that hand (without looking at it) gives no information concerning the sensory cortex. But if the primary sensations are normal in the hand, and the sensory information passes unaltered into the parietal lobe, then the inability to recognize an object in the hand indicates an abnormality of this lobe. Thus, the primary sensory modalities must be evaluated first.

There are many clinical tests that evaluate cortical sensory functions. All have in common the requirement that primary sensory information be integrated with memories regarding elemental properties such as texture, form, contour, weight, and temperature, and with previous experience in the recognition of tactile images. Motion and position sense, already mentioned, are ultimately cortical functions, assuming that the intervening pathways are intact.

Stereognosis, perception of the form and nature of an object through touch, is a sensitive and easily performed test. After asking the patient to close his eyes, the examiner places several familiar objects, one at a time, into each hand and the patient is asked to identify them. Similar information is obtained through the test of *graphesthesia.* Using a pointed object, the examiner writes two or three numbers on the palm or a fingertip of each hand, on the dorsum of each foot, and on other portions of the body if desired; but the numbers must be written larger in less sensitive areas. Normal persons can usually identify these familiar symbols.

Two-point discrimination is another valuable test. Two pointed objects, such as pins or the approximated ends of a paper clip, are simultaneously applied to the skin. The patient is asked whether he feels one or two stimuli. To assure reliability, a single point is occasionally applied. On the fingertips, a normal person can appreciate two separate points applied simultaneously when they are 3 to 4 mm. apart. At closer distances, the stimuli are interpreted as being a single point. This test is particularly important because it has a quantitative aspect; the number of millimeters of separation required for perception of two separate points is recorded, affording a basis for comparison with future tests.

Double simultaneous stimulation, the appreciation of two simultaneous touches or pinpricks, presented on symmetrically opposite areas of the body, requires normal cortical function. If only one is perceived, the parietal cortex on that side—that is, opposite the side of nonperception—may be abnormal. For valid test results, presentation of a single stimulus to the affected side must be perceived. The failure to recognize one of the stimuli is called *extinction* or *inattention.* The test may be very sensitive, revealing dysfunction when the sensory examination is otherwise normal.

Visual extinction is particularly sensitive. Two stimuli, such as moving fingers, are presented to the patient in the right and left halves of his visual field. Lack of perception of one of the moving fingers also indicates cortical sensory dysfunction and may be present when individual testing of the visual fields is normal.

The psychophysiologic basis of extinction is complex and forms a part of the patient's appreciation of his body image and its relation with the environment. Lesions of the parietal lobe which become more extensive, particularly those in the right hemisphere, may produce not only extinction but actual denial of any abnormality of that side (e.g., hemiparesis), or occasionally denial of the affected side as part of the body.

The perception of pain and temperature, at least in a crude fashion, does not require a normal parietal cortex. Crude pain perception is thought to come into consciousness in the thalamus; thus, lesions which destroy the cortex and subcortical white matter but which leave the thalamic region intact do not severely alter the perception of pain and temperature, though cortical sensory functions will be altered. Recognition of degree or quality of pain, however, probably does require the intact cortex. Vibratory sense, similarly, is not abolished by lesions involving the cortex, although its perception may be qualitatively different.

Clinicoanatomic Correlations

The anatomic interpretation of sensory loss aids in the localization of lesions in cases where the history and the findings from other portions of the neurologic examination do not yield sufficient information. If a person gives a history of injury to the arm in the region of the ulnar nerve, and shows weakness of the muscles innervated by that nerve, the sensory loss in the ulnar nerve distribution is simply confirmatory. But in many cases the facts are not so clear, and sensory disturbances may provide the best evidence.

Fibers carrying pain and temperature perception from the skin pass through cutaneous nerves, and fibers carrying deep pain travel with muscle and joint branches of peripheral nerves. Nuclei (cell bodies) of these nerve fibers are in the dorsal root ganglia. Their central processes pass into the spinal cord, then enter the dorsal horn where they synapse with the second neurons in the pathway. The processes of these neurons cross the midline at or near the level of entrance, beneath the central canal, to enter the opposite *lateral spinothalamic tract* (Fig. 23). This tract ascends in the spinal cord and passes through the medulla, pons, and midbrain, to end in the thalamus by synapsing with the third neuron. These final neurons then transmit information from the thalamus to the sensory cortex. A lesion involving the lateral

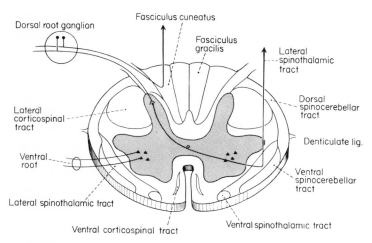

FIG. 23. Diagram of cross section of the spinal cord at cervical segment 7, showing major ascending and descending tracts and anterior horn cells.

spinothalamic tract will result in loss of pain and temperature sensation below the level of this lesion on the opposite side of the body.

Cell bodies of fibers conveying motion, position, and other discriminative sensations (two-point discrimination, stereognosis, and graphesthesia) as well as vibratory sense also lie in the dorsal root ganglia. The central processes enter the spinal cord and pass into the dorsal columns on the same side and then ascend to the medulla, where they synapse with the second neurons in the pathway. Their processes cross the midline in the lower medulla and ascend as the *medial lemniscus,* terminating in the thalamus. Fibers from the final neurons in this sequence project from the thalamus to the parietal cortex.

Simple touch sensation is carried by the *ventral spinothalamic tract,* which ascends to the thalamus after receiving both crossed and uncrossed fibers from the periphery. Discriminative touch sensation is also carried in the posterior columns. Since at least two pathways mediate perception of touch, it is rarely obliterated by spinal cord lesions unless the damage is severe. The perception of touch is often impaired by lesions of nerve roots and peripheral nerves, but almost always this loss is associated with the loss of other sensory modalities.

When multiple peripheral nerves are involved (*polyneuropathy;* see Chapter 3, "The Peripheral Nerves"), all modalities of sensation are reduced distally on the extremities; the legs are more severely affected than the arms. Perception of sensation gradually improves

as testing proceeds proximally. Sensory loss in lesions of single peripheral nerves corresponds to the distribution of the nerve. The medial,
ulnar, radial, femoral, sciatic, and common peroneal are the major
nerves affected by disease processes. The examiner must be familiar
with the motor, sensory, and reflex distribution of these nerves.

A lesion of a dorsal root produces loss of sensation in the segmental
distribution (*dermatome;* Fig. 24). Occasionally, objective loss may be
impossible to demonstrate (although the patient may describe it) since
there is considerable overlap peripherally between one dermatome and
another.

Lesions of a plexus cause a combination of nerve and root sensory
loss. Lesions of the brachial plexus are most common. If the upper
portion of the plexus is involved, the upper trunk and lateral cord
(cervical roots 5 and 6) are affected, resulting in weakness of shoulder
muscles and sensory loss in the region of the shoulder and lateral
border of the arm and forearm. A lower plexus lesion primarily affects
the lower trunk and medial cord (cervical root 8 and thoracic root 1)
causing weakness of the distal muscles of the arm, particularly the
intrinsic hand muscles, and sensory loss along the medial border of the
arm and forearm.

Two general patterns of sensory loss result from spinal cord lesions.
Hemisection of the cord (the *Brown-Sequard syndrome*) results in
loss of pain and temperature perception below the lesion on the opposite side and loss of proprioception below the lesion on the same side.
Voluntary motor activity is also lost on the same side, because of involvement of the corticospinal tract. The Brown-Sequard syndrome
usually results from lesions outside the spinal cord (extramedullary*)
which encroach upon it, but some intramedullary lesions also
produce it.

A lesion within the cord (intramedullary*) usually produces loss
of pain and temperature sensation in all dermatomes whose central
projections have been interrupted as they cross the midline. With such
lesions, touch sensation and proprioception are often preserved. *Dis-
sociation* of sensory loss, resulting in loss of pain but not touch, is
highly suggestive of an intramedullary lesion. These lesions most commonly occur in the cervical area of the spinal cord, and thus the pain
and temperature loss is detected in both upper extremities. In addition to this segmental loss, intramedullary lesions may extend to in-

---

* The terms *extramedullary* and *intramedullary* are derived from *medulla
spinalis,* an older term for the spinal cord. Curiously, they are used uncommonly
with reference to the *medulla oblongata.*

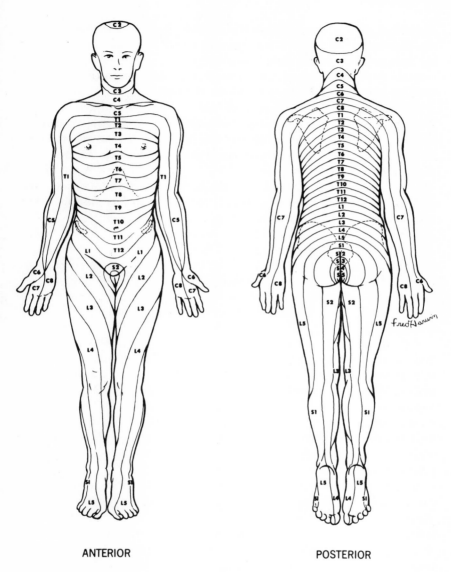

ANTERIOR   POSTERIOR

FIG. 24. Arrangement of dermatomes.

volve the spinothalamic pathways, causing loss of pain and temperature perception below the level of the lesion.

Lesions in the medulla and lower pons result in loss of pain and temperature sensation on the opposite side of the body, but on the same side of the face, because the entering pain fibers from the face via the trigeminal nerve descend as the spinal tract of the fifth nerve on the same side before they synapse.

Lesions from the upper pons, through the midbrain to the thalamus, produce contralateral loss of all forms of sensation.

Lesions of the thalamus, in addition to contralateral sensory loss, may also produce disagreeable spontaneous paresthesias, such as burning, itching, "electrical" sensations, and pain on the affected side of the body, usually initiated or aggravated by touching the skin.

Lesions of thalamocortical connections in the white matter of the cerebral hemispheres and of the parietal cortex generally spare the gross perception of vibration, pain, temperature, and crude touch, but result in cortical sensory loss.

Reflex activity is an important source of objective localizing information that is especially valuable because patient cooperation is not required to the extent necessary in other parts of the examination. In patients with lowered levels of consciousness, in whom more extensive neurologic evaluations are difficult, examination of the reflexes may afford the only localizing information. Alteration in reflexes may be the earliest sign of a disease involving the corticospinal or corticobulbar pathways (upper motor neuron), anterior horn cells or their axons (lower motor neuron), the sensory neurons from the muscles, or the muscles themselves.

For clinical purposes, reflexes are usually considered in three categories: (1) Muscle stretch reflexes, elicited by striking a tendon. Muscle stretch reflexes are also called *tendon reflexes, tendon jerks,* and, according to location, *knee jerk, ankle jerk,* and so on. These latter terms are brief and graphic, but they tend to suggest an incorrect physiologic basis for the muscle stretch reflex. (2) Cutaneous reflexes, elicited by stimulating the skin and observing a response in a related muscle group. Superficial reflexes have also been termed cutaneous reflexes. (3) Pathologic reflexes, obtainable only in the presence of disease. The most common and important pathologic reflexes are the Babinski and Chaddock signs.

Some of the important reflexes have been discussed in earlier sections. The *jaw reflex,* a typical muscle stretch reflex, and the *corneal reflex,* a superficial reflex, have been mentioned in connection with the trigeminal nerve. The *gag reflex,* mediated via the glossopharyngeal and vagus nerves, has also been discussed. The reflexes to be considered here are the clinically important muscle stretch reflexes in the extremities, significant cutaneous reflexes, and pathologic signs indicating a lesion of the corticospinal pathway.

Technique of Examination

MUSCLE STRETCH REFLEXES. In the arms, four muscle stretch reflexes are routinely elicited—biceps, triceps, brachioradialis, and finger flexor. Figure 25A–D illustrates the technique for obtaining each reflex, the spinal segments involved, and the peripheral nerves mediating the reflex.

To elicit the biceps reflex, place your thumb on the tendon of the patient's biceps muscle near its insertion to tense the muscle, then

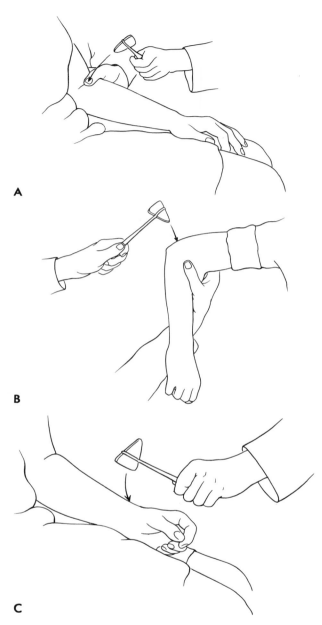

A

B

C

FIG. 25. Technique of obtaining muscle stretch reflexes. (A) Biceps reflex: C5, C6; musculocutaneous nerve. (B) Triceps reflex: C6–C8; radial nerve. (C) Brachioradialis reflex: C5, C6; radial nerve. (D) Finger flexion reflex: C7, C8; median and ulnar nerves. (E) Quadriceps reflex: L2–L4; femoral nerve. (F) Gastrocnemius reflex: S1; sciatic (tibial) nerve.

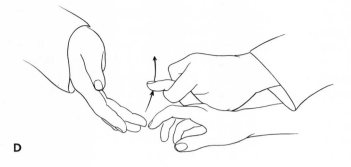

D

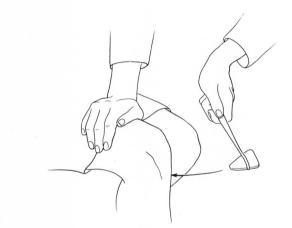

E

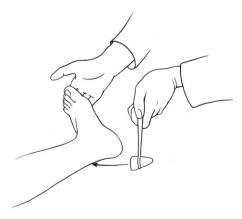

F

tap the thumb sharply with a reflex hammer with a slightly down-ward movement to enhance stretch of the muscle. The triceps and brachioradialis reflexes do not require tension exerted by the examiner's thumb, since these muscles are under adequate tension in the position illustrated. The finger flexor reflex (often called *Hoffman's sign*) is a muscle stretch reflex induced by tensing the flexor tendons of the middle finger by extending the metacarpophalangeal joint, then flicking the underside of the distal phalanx to produce a quick stretch. A positive response consists of quick flexion of the thumb and other fingers (see Fig. 25D). This reflex has the same significance as the other muscle stretch reflexes; however, normally the response is usually minimal or absent.

In the legs, two stretch reflexes are commonly tested (Fig. 25E, F). The quadriceps reflex is elicited by tapping the patellar tendon, the examiner's hand resting on the patient's quadriceps muscle. Thus, contraction of the quadriceps muscle can be felt even if no visible contraction occurs, as in a very obese patient. The "Achilles reflex" is obtained by placing the foot at a right angle to the leg, which tenses the gastrocnemius muscle, then striking its tendon.

Reflex responses among normal persons vary widely. The degree of reflex activity should be indicated in the patient's record by a grading system ranging from 0 to 4. Grade 1 is usually assigned to a minimal reflex response. Grades 2 and 3 are assigned to intermedi-ate reflex responses, depending on the examiner's judgment. Grade 4 indicates a very brisk reflex in which the muscle undergoes re-peated contractions, or *clonus*. Clonus is most frequently detected in the gastrocnemius. The examiner briskly dorsiflexes the patient's foot, sustaining the pressure, and notes any repetitive contractions of the muscle. Quick and sustained downward pressing on the patella may elicit clonus in the quadriceps muscle. A few beats of clonus may be found normally in individuals with brisk reflexes, but sustained clonus is abnormal, indicating a lesion of the upper motor neuron. Clonus at the wrist can occasionally be obtained by forceful dorsiflexion.

If muscle stretch reflexes cannot be elicited, *reinforcement techniques* should be used before concluding that the reflex is absent. Several methods are available. Perhaps the simplest is to ask the patient to contract minimally the muscle whose reflex is sought. With some muscles, such as the gastrocnemius, the patient may be able to do this simply by pressing his ankle lightly on the examiner's hand, which is placed on the ball of his sole. With other muscles, however, this is difficult—often too much pressure is exerted and the reflex becomes more difficult to elicit.

Another method of reinforcement consists of asking the patient to hook his fingers together and, on command, pull them in opposite directions while the examiner taps the tendon. This method is called the *Jendrassik maneuver*. A method to reinforce arm reflexes is to ask the patient to clench one fist tightly while the examiner simultaneously attempts to elicit a reflex in the opposite arm. All these maneuvers increase the facilitory activity of the spinal cord and thus accentuate minimally active reflexes. It is nearly always possible to elicit reflex responses in normal people if appropriate reinforcement techniques are carried out; the total absence of reflexes is rare in a normal person and requires explanation.

A cardinal principle in reflex evaluation is the comparison of each reflex on one side of the body with the corresponding reflex on the other side. Asymmetry may indicate the site of the suspected lesion. For example, upper motor neuron lesions in the brain cause accentuated muscle stretch reflexes on the opposite side because the corticospinal tract crosses the midline in the lower medulla; in the spinal cord, such lesions produce accentuated reflexes on the same side. Lower motor neuron lesions cause reduced reflex activity on the same side as the lesion.

The examiner must know the spinal cord segments and the peripheral nerves related to the major muscle stretch reflexes, as noted in Figure 25. When this information is added to other evidence from the examination and history, lesions can often be localized to a particular segment of the spinal cord or a peripheral nerve or nerve roots.

SUPERFICIAL REFLEXES. Two superficial reflexes are commonly tested, the abdominal and, in men, the cremasteric, which have in common an afferent arc from the skin to the cord as well as an efferent arc causing a muscular contraction. Both depend on an intact upper motor neuron pathway. If the lesion is above the decussation of the pyramids, the superficial reflexes will be absent on the opposite side of the body; if the lesion is below that level, the superficial reflexes will be absent on the same side as the lesion.

The superficial abdominal reflexes in the upper quadrants are mediated by segments T8 and T9; the lower, by T10 to T12. The reflexes are elicited by a light, rapid stroke on the skin of the abdomen in each upper and lower quadrant; the direction of the stroke is unimportant. The reflex may be obtained by a gentle scratch with a pin, key, pencil, or similar instrument. The normal response is a contraction of the superficial abdominal musculature. These reflexes are readily elicited in the average young person but may not be present in women who have had several pregnancies, in obese or elderly people, and in individuals who have had several abdominal operations. The response varies, however, even among normal people, and may be difficult to obtain, particularly if the abdomen is not relaxed.

In addition to aiding in the diagnosis of upper motor neuron lesions, these reflexes sometimes indicate the level of a spinal cord lesion. If, for example, the lower abdominal reflexes are absent but the upper preserved, the lesion may be between T9 and L1.

The cremasteric reflex is elicited by a stroke on the inner surface of the thigh. The normal response is a contraction of the cremaster muscle, which elevates the scrotum on that side. This reflex is easily obtained in most men and its absence on one side suggests the possibility of a corticospinal tract lesion.

The absence of these specific reflexes only very rarely occurs in the absence of other signs, and therefore they are of little practical importance in neurologic localization and diagnosis.

PATHOLOGIC REFLEXES. The *Babinski reflex* is sought by stroking the lateral border of the sole of the foot, beginning at the heel and moving toward the toes, carrying the stimulus across the ball of the foot toward the great toe. The stimulus should be firm but not painful. The instrument used may be a key, a pin, the end of a reflex hammer, or other pointed instrument. The normal response consists of flexion of all the toes, although in some normal persons there may be little or no reaction. The abnormal response—*Babinski sign*—consists of dorsiflexion of the great toe, sometimes with fanning of the other toes. Some avoid the eponym by speaking of *flexor* or *extensor plantar response,* for the normal or abnormal result, respectively (Fig. 26).

Difficulty may be encountered in distinguishing between a true Babinski sign and simple withdrawal of a sensitive or ticklish foot.

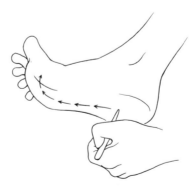

FIG. 26. Technique of eliciting the Babinski reflex. The sole is stroked firmly along the path indicated.

In such instances, a gentler stimulus should be used. This reflex is of great importance because it indicates a lesion of upper motor neuron pathways. In children under the age of 2, however, the reflex may be present normally.

When plantar responses produce equivocal results, a related reflex may be tested by stroking the lateral aspect of the dorsum of the foot from the heel toward the toes. Since this area is less sensitive than the sole, the reaction may be positive when the Babinski sign is difficult to evaluate. This is known as the *Chaddock sign,* and it is identical with the Babinski sign, both in significance and in the type of reaction —dorsiflexion of the great toe and fanning of the others. In a normal person, either there is no response or there is flexion of all the toes.

Numerous other ancillary tests with the same general significance have been described, and all are named for their describers. Only in rare instances are they helpful, the Babinski and Chaddock tests being sufficient in nearly all cases.

Clinicoanatomic Correlations

All muscle stretch reflexes consist of an afferent arc carrying impulses produced by the stretch of a muscle, a synapse within the spinal cord, and an efferent portion carrying impulses to the muscle. Interruption of this monosynaptic reflex arc by damage to any of its portions results in loss of the reflex (Fig. 27). A normal muscle stretch reflex also indicates that influences from higher centers modifying the reflex arcs are functioning. In the absence of these higher influences, the reflexes are abnormally vigorous and rapid, and elicited by a light tap on a tendon.

Such accentuation of the muscle stretch reflexes is of great diagnostic significance when it occurs on one side of the body, the reflexes on the other side being normal. The discrepancy suggests a disease of the

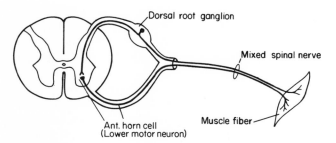

FIG. 27. Schematic view of a spinal reflex arc. The reflex will be lost if a lesion interrupts this arc at any point.

corticospinal tract related to the side of the body with the accentuated reflexes, and the likelihood is strengthened if a Babinski sign is demonstrated on the same side. If the muscle stretch reflexes are brisk on both sides of the body, the significance is less certain, because although it may indicate bilateral corticospinal tract disease, brisk reflexes are normal for some people. In such cases the Babinski sign is particularly important in the determination of abnormality of the corticospinal pathways.

Lesions of the upper motor neuron resulting in brisk reflexes include cerebrovascular occlusions and tumors of the cerebral hemispheres, and damage to the spinal cord from injuries and tumors. Degenerative and deficiency diseases, such as amyotrophic lateral sclerosis and pernicious anemia, may also involve the corticospinal pathways.

Lesions of the upper motor neuron pathways within the brain may lead to accentuation of all the muscle stretch reflexes in the opposite arm and leg, together with spasticity, weakness, and a Babinski sign on that side. Lesions in the spinal cord above the arm-related segments but below the decussation of the corticospinal tract in the caudal medulla will produce the same signs on the side of the lesion; lesions of the spinal cord in the thoracic or lumbar region produce the signs only in the affected leg.

Absence or diminution of the muscle stretch reflexes, especially in conjunction with wasting of the muscle, fasciculations, and weakness, indicates a lesion of the lower motor neuron. Diseases of the spinal cord which affect the anterior horn cells, such as poliomyelitis and amyotrophic lateral sclerosis, produce these findings. Similarly, the changes may be produced by tumors and injuries involving the gray matter of the anterior horn of the spinal cord; compression of the ventral roots of the spinal cord by tumors, injuries, or ruptured intervertebral discs; or peripheral nerve diseases.

Lesions of the sensory portion of the reflex arc also abolish the muscle stretch reflexes. In such instances, loss of sensation may be found in segments corresponding to the reflex loss. Examples include tabes dorsalis, a form of neurosyphilis affecting the dorsal roots and ganglia, and peripheral neuropathy, with damage to the sensory portions of peripheral nerves.

Diseases of the muscles, such as muscular dystrophy, also result in decreased or absent muscle stretch reflexes. Here the effect is due to loss or disease of muscle fibers rather than damage to the nerves that form the reflex arc.

NEUROLOGIC EXAMINATION OF INFANTS AND CHILDREN

The neurologic examination of a child differs in several important respects from that of an adult. In addition to the standard background information including the history and chief symptoms of the child's illness, the history of the mother's pregnancy and of the child's birth and development is of major interest to the examiner. Data concerning these periods may strongly suggest the diagnosis and may be of value in the ultimate prognosis.

In conducting the examination, emphasis centers on observation of the child's behavior and his responses to simple stimuli. Of great importance in a successful examination is a calm, relaxed, informal manner on the part of the examiner. It may be advisable for him to omit the traditional white coat.

INFANTS AND PRESCHOOL CHILDREN

In evaluating the infant or very young child, the physician should obtain the complete family history, including details of the birth and development of the child's siblings and of the mother's health record, with particular emphasis on such conditions as diabetes mellitus and other endocrine diseases, chronic renal disease, and drug intake, as well as the mother's possible exposure to radiation and infections during pregnancy. Other important facts concerning the pregnancy are threatened or attempted abortion, toxemia, and maternal injuries. The nature of the child's delivery should be ascertained in detail, including the duration of labor, anesthesia, the possibility of abruptio placentae, placenta praevia, induction of labor, Caesarian section, early rupture of membranes, breech delivery, and the necessity of resuscitation.

The duration of the pregnancy and the possibility of prematurity should be determined. An infant is termed premature if his period of gestation is less than 37 weeks or if he weighs less than 2,500 gm. Incidents occurring in the neonatal period, such as convulsions, lethargy, jaundice, poor feeding, excessive irritability, weak crying, and respiratory distress should be inquired about in detail. Signs like these, especially when combined with a history of slow development, strongly suggest brain damage.

The early feeding history of the child is important. The nature of his adaptation to bottle or breast, especially when compared to siblings, should be noted, as well as the rate of weight gain and increase in size in comparison with the standard percentile charts indicating weight and height increase with age.

The standard milestones should be carefully reviewed in the history as well as by observation during the examination. These include:

Age (months)	Activity
0–1	Lifts head when prone
4–5	Lifts head when supine, some full-hand grasping
7–8	Sits without support
9–10	Walks holding on, grasps with thumb and index finger
12–16	Walks unsupported

At 9 or 10 months of age, a child should understand a few words; at 10 or 12 months, he may use some words himself. By 24 months of age, he should be forming two- or three-word sentences.

Technique of Examination

The examiner should carefully observe the child during his spontaneous activity. On some occasions, it may be advisable to have the mother hold the child in her lap much of the time; on others, it may be rewarding simply to allow the child to move about the room at will. It is advisable not to undress the child immediately. Note should be made of the child's level of alertness and mood, and whether his general level of activity falls in the category of hyperactivity, excessive distractibility, restlessness, and irritability. The child's response to his parents and to the examiner may give clues to his psychologic development. Careful observation of the child's response to non-startling visual and auditory stimuli applied in a casual but systematic manner may provide information about his visual and auditory systems.

The general physical examination is an integral part of the neurologic assessment. It should include comparison of the head circumference with standard values, to determine whether microcephaly or macrocephaly is present. In infants, the skull should be transilluminated with a strong flashlight. Normally, only a 1 or 2 cm. red ring is visible. Larger red areas may indicate hydrocephalus, intracerebral cyst, or other fluid collections. The anterior fontanelle should be palpated. Normally it should be open, soft, and flat in infants. Distention indicates increased intracranial pressure, whereas a sunken fontanelle suggests dehydration.

The neck should be flexed for evidence of rigidity, an important sign in meningitis. Neck rigidity may be absent in very young infants with meningitis, however.

Inspection of the skin may reveal important diagnostic clues. Examples include the facial port-wine stain in Sturge-Weber disease, café-au-lait spots in neurofibromatosis, and depigmented nevi in tuberous sclerosis.

The physical development and symmetry of the limbs and spine should be noted. A variety of developmental malformations are manifested by abnormal configurations of the body, and may be associated with abnormalities of the nervous system.

Motor examination of the infant or young child can be assessed in large part by observing his manipulation of toys or other objects, and, if he is walking, the nature of his gait. Careful note should be made of asymmetry or marked preference for one hand or the other in a young child. Likewise, failure to grasp or maintain a hold with one arm or to kick or move one leg may be significant. Many of these observations can be facilitated by having a few attractive toys in strategic locations so that the child can react to them naturally.

The motor evaluation should be completed by some specific tests performed in a gentle and casual way. Muscle tone should be evaluated in all extremities, keeping in mind that normal infants have increased flexor tone generally, and that upper as well as lower motor neuron lesions produce hypotonia rather than spasticity in young children. A search for limitation of joint movement due to shortened muscle (contracture) in the major joints of the body should be carried out, as well as inspection of the musculature for atrophy. Abnormal postures should be noted. Strength of the extremities and trunk can be evaluated in several ways, including simply placing the child supine and having him roll over and stand up, observing the child's ability to pull himself up when offered help by the examiner's hand, and the ability to hold his head erect and steady. Significant lag of the head when the child is being pulled to a sitting from a supine position may indicate a pathologic condition if it persists beyond the age of 4 months.

The reflex examination in children can be carried out in a fashion similar to that in adults. Special care should be taken not to frighten the child with the reflex hammer. In infants the biceps and quadriceps reflexes are usually elicited readily. The grasp reflex of hands and feet as well as the sucking and rooting reflexes are normal in young infants. Reflex response to a sudden noise can give significant information regarding the brainstem pathways.

The Moro reflex, normal in young infants, should disappear between 15 and 20 weeks. It is elicited by holding the infant with his head supported in a slightly flexed position and then suddenly allowing the head to drop back about 30 degrees. The response should include sudden abduction and circumduction of the arms. The reflex should be symmetrical.

The tonic neck reflexes consist of extension of the ipsilateral arm when the child's head is forcibly turned to the side, together with flexion of the contralateral arm. These reflexes may be present in rudimentary form in infancy; if they are marked or persistent, a neurologic disorder is suggested.

The Landau reflex is evaluated by holding the infant in a prone position by supporting his abdomen. Normally, the head extends and the hips flex. If there is weakness of the lower extremities, hip flexion may not occur.

The plantar responses are normally extensor in infancy and may persist beyond the age of 1 year. Thus the Babinski sign, while of great importance in older children and adults, is of little help in neurologic evaluation in this age group.

Examination of the function of cranial nerves in infants is of necessity less detailed than in older children. The optic fundi should be inspected but it may be wise to defer this to the end of the examination, since it is upsetting to the child and will interfere with the remainder of the evaluation. Visual fields can be crudely evaluated by bringing objects in from the periphery and noting the point at which the infant turns his attention to them.

The function of the extraocular muscles may be evaluated by noting the spontaneous movements of the eyes, the turning of the infant's eyes in various directions in response to stimuli, such as a toy or a light, and the reflex eye movements when the head is suddenly moved toward one side or the other (doll's-eye movements). The pupillary reaction to light is tested and the presence of ptosis noted.

The trigeminal nerve may be evaluated by observing symmetry or asymmetry of jaw movements as the infant cries or talks, by palpation of the muscles of mastication, and by the response of the infant to pin and touch testing on the face.

Facial nerve function is assessed by watching the face during the infant's normal activity. Symmetry or asymmetry of facial musculature may be noted if the infant laughs or cries. A good estimate of facial and oropharyngeal coordination is obtained by observing the small infant suck from its bottle.

Hearing should be checked crudely by noting the response to various auditory stimuli; if hearing loss is suspected, formal tests including audiometry and other special measures should be carried out.

The glossopharyngeal and vagus nerves may be evaluated by noting the force and quality of the child's voice, the presence of nasality, hoarseness, and difficulty in swallowing.

The spinal accessory nerve is best tested by noting spontaneous muscle activity and by inspection and palpation of the sternocleidomastoid and trapezius muscles.

The hypoglossal nerve is evaluated by inspection of the tongue, noting its spontaneous movements, and searching particularly for fasciculations.

The sensory examination in an infant is difficult and usually not informative except in instances of severe spinal cord injury, where a level of sensory deficit can usually be demonstrated. Gross motor responses to pinpricks can usually be determined, but since these stimuli are unpleasant they should be deferred until the end of the examination. Evaluation of proprioception and cortical sensory mechanisms is impossible in infants.

OLDER CHILDREN

The examination of older children is like that of adults, except that it allows for the child's natural apprehension; the examination is adjusted so that stress is kept at a minimum. The procedures noted above concerning the general observation and behavior of the infant also apply in older children and are helpful in assessing the degree of development and adjustment to his environment.

The size and shape of the skull, including the status of the fontanelles, should be assessed and compared with standard charts. Similarly, measurements of height and weight, symmetry and quality of development of the limbs and spine, and assessment of the facial features and skin are important.

The technique of assessment of the mental status depends on the age of the child. The physician must be aware of the average mental capabilities of children of various ages. Simple tests for orientation and memory are available. The child's responses to requests to draw figures and pictures and to do simple arithmetic are assessed and a judgment made with respect to his overall level of activity and quality of behavior.

Frequently, the neurologic evaluation is performed for the purpose of assessing a learning or behavior problem; in such instances, evaluation of the mental status by a clinical psychologist is helpful. The physician, however, should assume the primary responsibility for detecting all illnesses, either neurologic or otherwise, which may be related to the difficulty in learning or abnormal behavior of the child.

Detailed examination of vision and hearing is essential. Methods vary, but with specialized techniques these functions may be assessed accurately even in young children. Speech impairment and speech patterns should be noted carefully, keeping in mind that the normal child has numerous pauses and hesitations in speech in the preschool and elementary school years. Performance in simple reading and auditory comprehension should be noted.

Examination of the cranial nerves proceeds in a manner analogous to that of an adult, again with care taken not to frighten or startle the child.

The motor examination can be more systematic in this age group, but it still depends largely on observation of spontaneous activity, as well as walking, hopping, skipping, and stair climbing, which often brings out subtle hip girdle weakness. Tests for strength and coordination can be carried out in the form of a pretended contest between the child and examiner. The muscle stretch reflexes and plantar responses should be elicited in the standard manner.

Sensory examination can be performed in more detail than in infancy, but it is still advisable to defer this until the end of the examination. The examination of pain perception should be brief, perhaps with demonstrations using the pin on the examiner's body first. Position and vibratory sense can be assessed in most older children if done with patience. Stereognosis may be assessed by asking the child to pick out an object from a group of small items without looking at them. Double simultaneous stimulation also can usually be carried out.

3   REGIONAL NEUROLOGIC DIAGNOSIS

THE CEREBRAL HEMISPHERES

The diseases that most frequently affect the cerebral hemispheres are primary and metastatic tumors, cerebral infarction and hemorrhage, penetrating head wounds, brain abscess, and congenital malformations. All these can produce similar signs on the neurologic examination, a fact that emphasizes the importance of the patient's history in the physician's diagnostic approach. Lesions of the hemispheres produce signs and symptoms in two ways. Negative symptoms are those which result from the destruction of a normally functioning area of the brain, for example, paralysis of the arm and leg on one side as the result of destruction of the motor cortex on the opposite side. Positive signs result from destruction of inhibitory areas, thus releasing activity not normally seen. An example of this is a movement disorder resulting from a disease of the basal ganglia.

The site of the lesion within the hemisphere obviously will determine the variety of signs produced. In addition to location, however, the rate of development of the disease is important in determining the clinical picture. Lesions which develop slowly, as for example a meningioma on the surface of the brain, may attain large size and yet produce only minimal signs. In addition, certain portions of the cerebral hemispheres are termed "silent" areas, because the localizing evidence for lesions here may be absent. The anterior portions of the frontal lobes and the right temporal lobe are examples. Slow-growing tumors in these regions may reach very large size without causing localizing neurologic signs.

The major symptoms caused by disease of the cerebral cortex concern higher-level integrative and interpretive motor and sensory functions, language, memory, intellect, and personality. Certain of these symptoms suggest a generalized bilateral disease and others focal or unilateral involvement.

The most important signs pointing specifically to the left cerebral hemisphere have to do with spoken and written language. Language functions are localized in the left hemisphere in most people regardless of handedness. In right-handed persons, language is always localized in the left cerebral hemisphere. In a few left-handed persons, the localization may be bilateral, and in some instances the function may be localized in the right cerebral hemisphere. For the most part, however, disturbance of language function, either writing or speaking (aphasia), suggests a cortical or subcortical lesion generally in the region of the left Sylvian fissure. The ability to perform fine, coordinated, learned acts with the hands and other parts of the body, a function called *praxis*, is also mainly localized in the left hemisphere. Defects in this function constitute *apraxia* (p. 18), and include inability to strike a match, manipulate a button, comb the hair, and perform other complex motor tasks, in the absence of weakness or sensory loss.

Certain complaints indicate involvement of both cerebral hemispheres. For example, loss of consciousness is generally thought to require abnormal function of both hemispheres. Consciousness may also be altered by lesions of the reticular formation in the mesencephalon and diencephalon. Intellectual deficits are much more profound when both hemispheres are involved, although they can be produced by unilateral lesions; this is also true of changes in behavior and personality. Impairment of motor and sensory functions on both sides of the body naturally implies that both cerebral hemispheres are involved. Such bilateral deficits, however, are common in brainstem and spinal cord diseases. Loss of control of the bladder, when due to hemisphere disease, suggests bilateral damage to the cerebral cortex in the region of the paracentral lobules.

THE FRONTAL LOBES

Either cortical or subcortical disease involving the anterior portion of the frontal lobes may result in personality and behavioral alterations and intellectual impairment. The patient may become apathetic or grandiose, irritable, suspicious, and hostile. No other neurologic signs may be present in early lesions.

If the lesion is in the posterior part of the frontal lobe, involving the motor area, contralateral monoparesis or hemiparesis results. If only a part of the motor cortex is affected, the impairment is localized, as for example isolated facial, leg, or arm weakness of upper motor neuron type. Motor dysfunction more often takes the form of hemiplegia or hemiparesis when the lesion is subcortical.

If the lesion is in the medial portion of the frontal lobe, anterior to the motor strip, reflex grasping movements of the opposite hand may occur when the examiner strokes his fingers against the patient's palm and fingers. However, the grasp reflex is most commonly detected bilaterally in patients with diffuse brain disease and dementia, and is of little importance in precise clinical localization.

Irritation of the frontal lobe eye fields (area 8) causes deviation of the eyes and head toward the opposite side, but when there is destruction of this area the deviation is toward the side of the lesion.

A lesion in the left frontal lobe in the inferior frontal gyrus posteriorly (Broca's area; see Fig. 1) may result in expressive or nonfluent aphasia.

Irritation in the motor area, such as that caused by a meningioma, results in focal or Jacksonian seizures which, if they remain localized, do not produce loss of consciousness.

THE PARIETAL LOBES

Disorders affecting either parietal lobe produce contralateral cortical sensory deficits, such as impairment of motion and position sense, two-point discrimination, localization of stimuli applied to various parts of the body, recognition of written symbols on the skin, and stereognosis. With cortical lesions, crude pain, temperature, touch, and vibratory perception is generally intact, but if the lesion is deep, particularly when it affects the thalamus, there may be profound loss of these modalities. A patient with a parietal lobe lesion may complain of numbness or unusual sensations on the opposite side of the body. It is not uncommon for the patient to note difficulty in recognizing coins or other objects in his pocket. Irritative lesions may results in sensory seizures consisting of episodic numbness and tingling or other odd sensations on the contralateral side of the body.

A psychologic function called *body imagery* is localized to the parietal lobes. A lesion in the right lobe distorts the patient's awareness of the left side of his body; he may deny that there is impairment of function on that side, or even that the left side exists at all. If asked to draw the face of a clock or the petals on a flower, he may draw half the figure accurately but ignore or distort the other (contralateral to the affected lobe). The failure to appreciate double simultaneous stimulation—*extinction*—is usually the initial manifestation of disturbance of body imagery (see p. 73).

An interesting phenomenon called *constructional apraxia* occurs with lesions of the parietal lobes. The patient's inability to reproduce or conceptualize three-dimensional objects or pictures signifies a primary defect in the ability to perceive spatial relationships in the environment. A simple test is to ask the patient to copy a cube that you draw for him. Disturbance in both body imagery and apraxia are most easily evaluated in lesions of the nondominant hemisphere because aphasia usually interferes with testing when the dominant hemisphere is affected.

Since the visual radiations are located, in part, in the deep white matter beneath the parietal cortex, deep lesions may cause characteristic defects in the fields of vision. The most common defect is an homonymous hemianopia, but with less extensive lesions; there may be an homonymous defect in the inferior quadrant, on the side opposite the parietal lobe lesion.

THE TEMPORAL LOBES

A unique group of seizures is among the important manifestations of temporal lobe lesions. Diseases of the temporal cortex in the region of the uncus or hippocampal gyrus on either side (see Fig. 2) may produce olfactory hallucinations, sometimes accompanied by smacking of the lips and alteration of consciousness. Other irritative phenomena characteristic of temporal lobe seizures include auditory and formed visual hallucinations, déjà vu, dreamy states, and psychomotor seizures, described on page 99.

Since the majority of the visual radiations lie in the temporal lobes, defects in the field of vision are common. Complete homonymous hemianopia on the opposite side is most common, but if the lesion is small and remains localized to the temporal lobe, an homonymous superior quadrant field defect may be produced.

If the lesion is in the left temporal cortex, aphasia of predominantly fluent or receptive type may occur, accompanied by auditory agnosia.

THE OCCIPITAL LOBES

Lesions involving the occipital lobe in the region of the calcarine fissure (area 17) produce homonymous hemianopia on the opposite side which spares the macular area. The visual field defects in the two eyes are of the same configuration—that is to say, they are congruent. If the lesion is in area **18** or **19** in the dominant hemisphere, difficulty in visual object recognition (visual agnosia) and reading comprehension (alexia) may develop, since these areas lie adjacent to temporal and parietal association regions important in visual interpretations. Irritative lesions of the occipital lobes may result in seizures preceded by a visual aura consisting of poorly formed lights, colors, and shapes.

LOCALIZING ASPECTS OF CONVULSIVE DISORDERS

Convulsive disorders (epilepsy) are manifestations of a wide variety of neurologic and systemic illnesses. In some cases, convulsive seizures have focal aspects which aid in topographic neurologic diagnosis, and they are considered from that standpoint here.

Seizures result from poorly understood physicochemical changes in brain cells. Their frequency is highly variable. They may occur several times each day, or a patient may have only one in his lifetime. The central event in a seizure is an uncontrolled discharge of neurons, with resulting psychic, behavioral, motor, sensory, or autonomic manifestations. Among the known causes are birth injury, tumor, trauma, infection, toxins, and metabolic disturbances. In many patients, however, the cause cannot be determined (idiopathic epilepsy).

Since the physician usually does not observe the seizure, the history is the major source of information regarding the type and cause of the episodes. It should include prenatal and perinatal events, the immediate postnatal period, and early mental and physical development; and the physician should search for complaints suggesting one of the known causes.

One of the major historical points is a description of an *aura* preceding the actual seizure. The aura is often regarded as a warning, or a prodrome, to a seizure, but it is actually an integral part of the attack. It is usually brief, lasting seconds to minutes. A strange epigastric sensation is a common aura of limited localizing value. It may ascend to the head or spread diffusely. The aura may include phenomena of localizing value, however, and should be carefully described. For example, it may consist of sensory complaints such as numbness, suggesting parietal lobe origin. Visual phenomena, for example colors or lights, suggest occipital localization.

GRAND MAL SEIZURES

These are the most common variety. They may begin with an aura, then abrupt loss of consciousness, sometimes preceded by an involuntary cry. Tonic contraction of trunk and extremity muscles occurs, often of great intensity, followed by clonic jerking movements of the extremities, the trunk, and the jaw. During the tonic phase the patient is apneic and may become cyanotic. Incontinence of bowel and bladder is common. The tongue is often bitten. The duration of the seizure varies from one to several minutes. A postseizure (postictal) state of confusion, headache, and fatigue may last for several hours. The patient often sleeps during this period. Following treatment with anticonvulsants such as phenobarbital, grand mal seizures may be manifested by only loss of consciousness for a few seconds. These seizures are then frequently, but erroneously, diagnosed as petit mal but are properly termed abortive grand mal seizures.

The grand mal seizure itself is nonspecific for localization, but the aura preceding it is often of major localizing value. Occasionally transient postseizure weakness on one side of the body (Todd's paralysis) localizes the lesion to the opposite hemisphere.

JACKSONIAN SEIZURES

Jacksonian seizures* are major convulsions of localizing significance. A movement, usually clonic, begins in one portion of the body, for example the thumb or fingers, and spreads to involve the wrist, arm, face, and leg on one side (Jacksonian march). Such a focal seizure may cease at any point or spread to involve the opposite side of the body with resulting loss of consciousness and a grand mal seizure. These seizures indicate an abnormal area in the motor cortex of the opposite hemisphere. Todd's paralysis may occur after the attack.

Occasionally, a focal seizure with a sensory march occurs, similar to the motor march. Such seizures indicate an abnormality in the opposite parietal cortex.

PETIT MAL SEIZURES

These are minor seizures which occur in children and rarely in adults. In a typical petit mal attack there is a period of altered consciousness, lasting only a few seconds, during which the child pauses and stares. Motor movements, if present at all, consist of slight nodding

---

* After Hughlings Jackson, the English neurologist who first described these attacks.

of the head or blinking. The patient is unaware of what transpires during the attacks. If the seizures occur many times each day, as petit mal often does, the child may have difficulty comprehending schoolwork and erroneously be judged a "daydreamer" or retarded. The electroencephalogram shows a characteristic three-per-second spike-wave pattern (see Fig. 38). These attacks usually decrease as the patient approaches adulthood, but grand mal seizures develop in a high proportion of cases.

AKINETIC SEIZURES

These seizures may be related to petit mal because of similarities in the EEG patterns. In these attacks, the individual suddenly falls to the ground with or without loss of consciousness. Within a moment or two the seizure ends and he is able to rise and pursue ordinary activities. Neither akinetic nor petit mal seizures have localizing value from a practical standpoint. They are thought to originate in the deep nuclear masses of the diencephalon.

MYOCLONIC SEIZURES

These seizures consist of jerking movements of one or more extremities. For example, a jerk or two of flexion at the elbow may constitute a seizure. They may or may not be symmetrical. Such seizures occur mainly in the morning and, if unassociated with other types of seizures, are termed *benign morning myoclonus.*

Myoclonic seizures not uncommonly occur in patients who also have grand mal seizures. They also occur in several serious degenerative diseases, particularly in children.

TEMPORAL LOBE SEIZURES

In addition to areas relating to language, memory, and hearing, numerous psychic and behavioral phenomena are related to temporal lobe structures. When seizures result from temporal lobe lesions, therefore, a wide variety of manifestations may occur.

PSYCHOMOTOR SEIZURES. During these episodes, which usually occur without warning, the patient enters a dissociated state of consciousness (dreamy state) in which he carries out inappropriate or, at times, appropriate actions for which he is amnesic. Behavior may range from irrelevant movements of the extremities to attacks of rage. Many times the patient continues to carry out seemingly purposeful activity—for example, a patient walking home may suddenly lose "ordinary" consciousness, yet find himself in his home without remembering anything about the last few blocks of his trip. Such seizures usually last from a few minutes to 20 or 30 minutes; if they are prolonged, they must be differentiated from fugue states of psychiatric origin.

DÉJÀ VU.   These are attacks of impaired consciousness during which the patient has a vivid, dreamlike impression that the situation he is in at the moment is a precise repetition of a previous experience. Sometimes the impression is the opposite—that a familiar situation has suddenly become totally strange (jamais vu). The attacks are momentary but very "real" to the patient.

VISUAL HALLUCINATIONS.   These may occur as a form of temporal lobe seizure. Since the posterior portions of the temporal lobes are adjacent to visual association areas, these seizures may include formed visual hallucinations, such as people, animals, landscapes, and other familiar sights. In some cases, however, the vision is distorted in some way. For example, the persons he sees may be tiny (micropia), large (macropia), or deformed, or have an unusual color or appearance.

AUDITORY HALLUCINATIONS.   Irritation of the auditory association areas result in attacks in which perception of voices, music, or strange noises may occur.

UNCINATE SEIZURES.   These result from lesions of the uncus, a portion of the medial temporal lobe. Because olfactory and gustatory areas are located (in part) within the temporal lobe, hallucinations of smell and taste may develop, often associated with smacking of the lips and tasting movements of the tongue.

Many of these attacks suggest psychiatric disorders. Their organic nature is determined by the fact that they are brief, episodic, and stereotyped, and occur in individuals without other signs or history of mental disease. The differential diagnosis may be difficult if the patient with organic seizures happens to have a history of a serious personality disorder.

THE BASAL GANGLIA AND EXTRAPYRAMIDAL SYSTEM

The basal ganglia include the caudate nucleus, putamen, globus pallidus, and amygdala (Figs. 28, 29, 30). The amygdala has olfactory and hypothalamic connections. The olfactory functions are probably insignificant in man. The amygdala probably functions in relation to the visceral responses to emotional stimuli. There are no specific clinical findings that allow localization of a lesion to this structure.

In addition to these structures, the substantia nigra, subthalamic nucleus, red nucleus, and brainstem reticular formation are usually

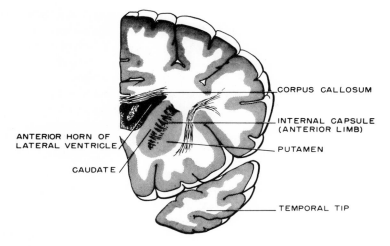

FIG. 28. Coronal section of right hemisphere through level of head of caudate nucleus.

considered to be closely related functionally, and they form, collectively, the major part of the *extrapyramidal motor system*. These regions are closely interrelated by fiber tracts; in addition, fibers to and from the cerebral cortex and projections to the lower motor neurons of the brainstem and spinal cord are included within this system.

Although the extrapyramidal system is the major motor pathway in lower life forms, the appearance of a highly developed corticospinal

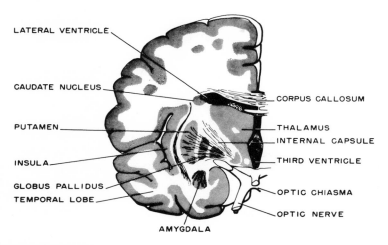

FIG. 29. Coronal section of right hemisphere through level of globus pallidus.

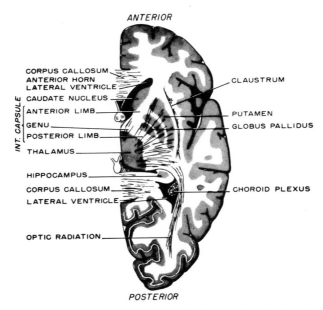

FIG. 30. Horizontal section of right hemisphere through level of internal capsule.

system in man has relegated it to a subordinate, though still important, role. The extrapyramidal motor system probably is important in maintaining posture and postural adjustments and in the grosser volitional movements, particularly of proximal joints, to form a steadying and reinforcing influence for superimposed finely coordinated movements which are mediated by the corticospinal system. Through complex interrelationships between the extrapyramidal motor structures, the corticospinal and corticobulbar systems, and the cerebellum, the highly developed volitional movement patterns of man are achieved.

Clinically, lesions involving the extrapyramidal system produce two varieties of symptoms. An increase in muscle tone, termed *rigidity*, sometimes associated with slowness (*bradykinesia*) of voluntary movements develops on the side of the body opposite a lesion. If lesions are bilateral, and rigidity is widespread, the patient stands and walks with a posture of generalized flexion. Various movement disorders also occur in diseases of the extrapyramidal system: tremors, chorea, athetosis, dystonia, and ballism, all described in Chapter 2. Abnormal movements occur on the side opposite a lesion.

The correlation of a specific movement disorder with specific lesions within the basal ganglia is not always possible. Parkinsonism, characterized clinically by tremor, bradykinesia, and rigidity, is characterized pathologically by lesions that are most severe in the substantia nigra but that also affect the globus pallidus and other structures.

Athetosis probably results from damage to putamen and caudate nuclei and related structures. This entity is usually the result of injury to the brain from prenatal and natal factors.

Huntington's chorea, a chronic progressive disease inherited in autosomal dominant fashion, is characterized by severe damage to the putamen and caudate nuclei and the cerebral cortex, resulting in gross choreic movements as well as dementia.

Ballism or hemiballism is more specifically related to malfunction of a single structure, the subthalamic nucleus. The damage usually results from vascular occlusion.

Wilson's disease, a disorder of copper metabolism, is characterized clinically by tremor, dystonia, and athetosis, as well as liver disease. Severe lesions are found in the globus pallidus, but other portions of the basal ganglia are affected as well.

Although the basal ganglia are affected, the pathophysiologic alterations necessary for the development of dystonia are not known.

THE PITUITARY REGION

Of the lesions that develop in this area, pituitary adenoma has the highest incidence. Lesions that should be differentiated from pituitary adenoma include meningioma of the tuberculum sellae, aneurysm in the siphon of the internal carotid artery, glioma of the optic nerve, and craniopharyngioma.

Defects in the visual fields and impairment of visual acuity are frequently noted (see Fig. 6). Any suspicion of a lesion in the pituitary area should lead to careful visual field testing by means of confrontation and tangent screen examination. The visual abnormality is usually a bitemporal hemianopia which in most cases begins in the upper quadrants; however, the nature of the visual defects will vary according to the location and behavior of the lesion. Anterior lesions such as optic nerve glioma may destroy one optic nerve while sparing the other. Lesions posterior to the chiasm in the optic tracts may cause homonymous hemianopia. Lesions in the pituitary region may result in complete blindness. During the early stages, the patient may be unaware of the development of visual deficits.

Pituitary tumors cause various disturbances in endocrine functions that are normally under the control of pituitary hormones. Tumors which destroy normal pituitary tissue, such as chromophobe adenoma, may result in hypothyroidism, hypoadrenalism, and hypogonadism. The earliest evidence of pituitary dysfunction in women is a change in the pattern of the menstrual periods, usually amenorrhea. In men, impotence and loss of body hair may be noticed first. Decrease in frequency of shaving is reported; occasionally it is discovered that the patient has never shaved more than once or twice a week.

Impaired function of the thyroid gland is manifested by symptoms of hypothyroidism, such as dry and finely wrinkled skin, loss of hair, intolerance to cold, and fatigue and lethargy. Reduced adrenal function also contributes to fatigue, and in addition causes abnormal pigmentation of the skin and lowered resistance to infection.

Tumors of the eosinophilic cells of the pituitary gland produce the clinical syndrome of *acromegaly*, characterized by overgrowth of bony and soft tissues throughout the body. The effects are particularly noticeable in the face, where enlargement of the mandible, frontal bones, and soft tissue occurs. Enlargement of the hands may become noticeable first when rings become too tight.

Hyperfunction or hypofunction of the pituitary gland before puberty may result in gigantism or dwarfism, respectively.

Craniopharyngioma presents special diagnostic and therapeutic problems. The lesion occurs much more often in children than in adults. In the child, the lesion is usually calcified and the diagnosis may be suspected from plain x-rays of the skull; in adults, however, calcification is less common. Craniopharyngiomas develop in the suprasellar region. Because of the proximity of these tumors to the optic chiasm, they may affect the fields of vision, and they have been known to grow so large as to destroy the visual pathways and cause total blindness. Their proximity to hypothalamic structures means that children so affected may experience retardation of growth and development, including the secondary sexual characteristics. When the posterior lobe of the pituitary or its hypothalamic connections are involved, the lack of antidiuretic hormone may result in diabetes insipidus. Characteristic are polyuria, intense thirst, and very dilute urine, of a specific gravity less than 1.010.

Surgical operations in the hypothalamic region often produce severe disturbance in hypothalamic functions, and the postoperative management of such patients is complex.

Tumors in the pituitary region do not commonly produce signs of increased intracranial pressure. Occasionally, however, such a tumor reaches sufficient size to obstruct the flow of cerebrospinal fluid through the third ventricle, resulting in a rise in pressure.

THE THIRD VENTRICLE AND MIDBRAIN

The most important lesions in this area are tumors and cysts in the posterior portion of the third ventricle, the upper part of the midbrain, and the pineal gland. In addition, occlusion of blood vessels supplying the midbrain is sometimes noted. The effects of disease in this region include increased intracranial pressure, altered consciousness, oculomotor abnormalities, and motor dysfunction. Because of the small caliber of the aqueduct of Sylvius, small lesions can completely obstruct the flow of cerebrospinal fluid and cause an increase in intracranial pressure before localizing signs and symptoms develop. Also, the aqueduct may be obstructed at its origin by tumors, usually gliomas, extending into it from structures adjacent to the third ventricle.

Since the oculomotor nerve nuclei and their connections are in this area, abnormal extraocular movements may provide localizing evidence. A lesion causing pressure on the superior colliculi, such as a pineal gland tumor, usually results in early impairment of conjugate upward gaze (Parinaud's syndrome); dilated pupils and impairment of downward gaze are noted later.

Lesions involving the efferent fibers from the oculomotor nerve nuclei on one side, as well as the corticospinal tract fibers in the cerebral peduncle adjacent to the nerve, produce *Weber's syndrome*, which consists of ipsilateral oculomotor nerve palsy with contralateral hemiparesis (see Fig. 14).

With the rapid expansion of a supratentorial lesion such as an epidural hematoma, the upper portion of the midbrain may be compressed by the medial part of the ipsilateral temporal lobe. The resultant involvement of the ipsilateral oculomotor nerve is signaled by dilatation of the pupil, followed by signs of bilateral involvement of the corticospinal tract. Compression of the reticular formation in the midbrain causes alteration of consciousness. These midbrain signs indicate that surgery must be performed at once to relieve the pressure.

THE CEREBELLUM

Cerebellar dysfunction frequently results from primary and metastatic tumors, demyelinating diseases, and various drugs and toxins. Other diseases affecting this area include abscess, encephalitis, trauma, and certain genetically determined states such as the spinocerebellar degenerations. Lesions of the cerebellum cause signs following three general patterns which can be correlated with the functional anatomy of the cerebellum.

The cerebellar hemispheres and the midline structures (see Figs. 3, 14) are the important subdivisions of the cerebellum for clinical correlations. The cerebellar hemispheres are newer phylogenetically and are related to the massive development of the cerebral cortex in man. The cerebellar hemispheres regulate motor activities requiring control and modulation, such as fine coordinated movements of fingers. Each cerebellar hemisphere is related to the opposite motor cortex, since the projection paths from the cerebellum to the cerebral cortex cross in the brachium conjunctivum. But since the projection fibers from the cortex also cross the midline, a lesion of one cerebellar hemisphere will result in dysfunction of the arm and leg on the same side.

Physical examination reveals hypotonia, difficulty in performing rapid alternating movements, and impairment of rhythm and co-ordination in the finger-nose, heel-shin, and similar tests. The gait is ataxic and the patient tends to fall toward the abnormal side. Nystagmus may occur, most marked when the patient looks toward the side of the lesion.

The midline structures of the cerebellum, termed the *vermis*, are older phylogenetically and are primarily concerned with coordination of axial musculature. The projection fibers from the vermis follow the same general pattern as those from the cerebellar hemispheres but act to influence truncal musculature and walking. Lesions of the vermis produce gait ataxia resulting in a wide-based, staggering, uneven gait, and a tendency to fall toward either side. Ataxia of the trunk muscles may be apparent if the patient sits unsupported. The examiner may note irregular jerky movements of the trunk and neck as the patient attempts to maintain his balance.

Cerebellar hemisphere and vermis syndromes often overlap; for example, a tumor that arises in a cerebellar hemisphere produces its characteristic syndrome and may then extend to the vermis to produce truncal ataxia as well.

An important pattern of cerebellar dysfunction results from diffuse involvement by drugs and toxins, such as sedatives, diphenylhydan-toin, and alcohol, and also by diffuse infection (encephalitis). Generalized ataxia may develop, involving trunk, extremities, gait, and speech. Nystagmus is often present. Since intoxication with various drugs and alcohol is common, this diffuse picture of cerebellar dysfunction is the most frequent type seen clinically.

THE PONS AND MEDULLA

When these regions are affected, a combination of cranial nerve impairment and motor and sensory abnormalities of the arms and legs ("long tract signs") develop. An example of such a lesion is thrombosis of the posterior inferior cerebellar artery (*Wallenberg's syndrome*) causing infarction of the lateral superior aspect of the medulla (see Fig. 14). The syndrome reflects damage to the trigeminal, acoustic, glossopharyngeal, and vagus nerve nuclei, the cerebellar connections, the reticulospinal pathways, and the spinothalamic tract, resulting in:

1. Loss of pain and temperature perception on the ipsilateral side of the face because of involvement of the spinal tract and nucleus of the trigeminal nerve
2. Loss of pain and temperature perception on the contralateral side of the body because of involvement of the lateral spinothalamic tract
3. Ataxia of the arm and leg on the side of the lesion because of damage to the inferior cerebellar peduncle
4. Vertigo and nystagmus because of involvement of the vestibular nuclei and their connections
5. Paresis of the palate and impaired gag reflex on the side of the lesion, and hoarseness and dysphagia because of involvement of the nucleus ambiguus (glossopharyngeal and vagus nerves)
6. Horner's syndrome on the side of the lesion because of damage to the reticulospinal pathway

Structures near the midline of the medulla, such as the medial lemniscus, the corticospinal pathway, and the hypoglossal nerve and nucleus, are spared in this syndrome since the involved artery does not supply the midline structures.

The brainstem glioma, a slow-growing tumor occurring primarily in children, is another common lesion within the substance of the pons and medulla. The signs and symptoms indicate bilateral involvement of the brainstem, which is in contrast to Wallenberg's syndrome. Most commonly the abducens and facial nerves and their nuclei are affected, producing diplopia and facial weakness. These tumors usually involve the corticospinal pathways, causing spasticity and paresis of the arms and legs and gait disturbances. As the tumor expands, other cranial nerves, for example the glossopharyngeal and vagus nerves, are damaged, with resulting dysarthria and dysphagia.

Lesions adjacent to the brainstem which infringe on it and involve emerging cranial nerves are relatively frequent. The most important is the acoustic neuroma (see p. 51), a tumor arising on the acoustic nerve at its entrance into the internal acoustic meatus of the temporal bone. The early symptoms of these tumors are reduced hearing and tinnitus, a ringing or rushing sound in the affected ear. These symptoms develop insidiously and may be minimal for many months. Tinnitus, particularly, may be present for only a few months and then disappear, and hearing loss may be unnoticed since the person has normal hearing in the opposite ear. As the tumor expands, however, it begins to encroach upon adjacent structures such as the trigeminal nerve, resulting in a reduced corneal reflex and sensory loss on the face. Still later, the tumor compresses the inferior cerebellar peduncle and cerebellum, and this results in ataxia of the ipsilateral arm and leg. In some cases, these tumors descend in the posterior fossa and involve the glossopharyngeal, vagus, and spinal accessory nerves. Curiously, despite its proximity to the acoustic nerve, the facial nerve is usually not affected until the tumor is large.

If a tumor, such as a medulloblastoma arising from midline cerebellar structures, or an ependymoma arising from ependymal cells in the ventricle, obstructs flow of cerebrospinal fluid through the fourth ventricle, a characteristic clinical picture occurs. Unsteadiness of gait develops because of involvement of the vermis of the cerebellum in the roof of the fourth ventricle. Abrupt vomiting, sometimes without nausea, occurs because of damage to the floor of the fourth ventricle, which contains vagal nuclei and other centers controlling gastric function. Headache, lateral rectus muscle weakness with diplopia, and papilledema develop because of rising intracranial pressure. If the lesion is not treated, there will be obtundation, alterations in vital signs, and episodes of unconsciousness, indicating grave compromise of vital centers.

Intermittent insufficiency of blood flow through the vertebrobasilar arterial system produces the syndrome of basilar artery insufficiency. Brief episodes of dysfunction of brainstem structures occur in random sequence and pattern. Diplopia, vertigo, dysarthria, numbness of the face or of either side of the body, gait ataxia, and hemiparesis are examples. Visual symptoms, such as blurring, transient blindness, and field defects occur because portions of the visual pathways are supplied by the posterior cerebral arteries, the terminal branches of the basilar artery. Symptoms rarely last more than a few minutes and then clear completely.

Complete occlusion of the basilar artery produces quadriplegia, diffuse sensory loss, extraocular muscle palsies, facial weakness, dysarthria, dysphagia, and altered consciousness. The prognosis is grave and most patients die within a few days.

Diseases affecting motor portions of medullary cranial nerve nuclei, such as poliomyelitis, result in bulbar palsy, which has been described on page 53.

INCREASED INTRACRANIAL PRESSURE

Regardless of its cause, increased intracranial pressure in itself produces a group of signs and symptoms of great importance. Papilledema is the most important sign of increased intracranial pressure (see p. 27). It results from obstruction of venous return from the eyeball, caused by elevated pressure in the cerebrospinal fluid around the optic nerve. Papilledema develops within a day or two after intracranial pressure begins to rise; it will not be found in the first few hours of such a rise, however.

Headache is the most common symptom. The pain varies in location and severity but is especially intense in those patients whose intracranial pressure is rising rapidly. Maneuvers which normally increase intracranial pressure, such as straining, coughing, or sneezing, increase the severity of the headache. The pain is usually worse following sleep or recumbency, and lessens somewhat during the day. There is no characteristic site of pain; usually it is generalized.

Stiff neck may occur, particularly if the rise in pressure is rapid. It is more frequent in posterior fossa tumors, but may be seen with mass lesions anywhere in the cranium. It may be associated with herniation of the temporal lobe through the tentorial notch (tentorial pressure cone, p. 105). Stiff neck also may be found when the tonsils of the cerebellum herniate through the foramen magnum; this serious situation is most likely to occur in patients with posterior fossa tumors.

Vomiting, sometimes of a violent or projectile type, is associated with the increased pressure, particularly if there are lesions affecting the structures in the posterior cranial fossa, because of the proximity of centers related to visceral function. Increased pressure from any cause, however, may cause vomiting, with or without nausea.

Periodic fluctuation in consciousness with the gradual development of drowsiness and stupor is characteristic of increasing pressure, presumably because of involvement of the reticular formation and related structures. If the rise is rapid, coma may occur rapidly.

As intracranial pressure rises, pulse rate falls. This typical sign is valuable in following the course of a patient with a suspected intracranial mass lesion. Coincident with the fall in pulse, rising blood pressure is common, thus providing another warning. Respiration may be disturbed, with periods of normal or accelerated breathing alternating with periods when it slows or stops.

Certain false localizing signs may develop with increased intracranial pressure which suggest a lesion in a particular region of the brain but actually indicate the effects of mechanical forces produced by the pressure. For example, abducens nerve palsy in such cases results from the stretching and distortion of this long intracranial nerve simply by pressure. The result is paresis of the lateral rectus muscle, usually affecting one side but sometimes both sides. Therefore, abducens nerve palsy in the presence of increased intracranial pressure is not necessarily a localizing sign.

A much less frequent false sign is the development of hemiplegia ipsilateral to an expanding supratentorial mass, which results from compression of the opposite cerebral peduncle against the tentorium. Another example, interesting but rare, is bitemporal hemianopia resulting from pressure on the optic chiasm through dilatation of the third ventricle. The dilatation may be caused by obstruction of cerebrospinal fluid flow in the posterior third ventricle, the aqueduct, or the fourth ventricle.

THE SPINAL CORD

Lesions affecting the spinal cord produce a combination of *segmental* (horizontal) *signs*—lower motor neuron signs, dermatome sensory loss, reflex depression or loss—and *long tract* (vertical) *signs*—dorsal columns, lateral spinothalamic tract, corticospinal tract—which usually allow accurate localization. Such localization requires knowledge of the anatomy of the spinal cord, including the motor and sensory tracts, and the motor, sensory, and reflex patterns of the various segments.

Lesions occurring within the substance of the spinal cord are termed *intramedullary* and include primary tumors such as ependymomas and gliomas, and hemorrhages, arteriovenous malformations, and congenital cavities such as syringomyelia. Lesions occurring outside the spinal cord but within the confines of the dura are termed *extramedullary intradural*, and the most common of these are meningiomas (especially in women) and neurofibromas. Lesions occurring outside the dura are called *extramedullary extradural*. Examples of extradural lesions are herniated intervertebral discs, metastatic tumors, and epidural abscesses.

The clinical findings in intramedullary lesions consist of segmental motor, sensory, and reflex disturbances, usually bilateral, together with signs of involvement of the long ascending and descending tracts in the spinal cord. Because these intramedullary lesions commonly interrupt the axons carrying pain and temperature sensation in the center of the cord where they cross, the resulting sensory loss is bilateral and extends throughout the segments involved in the lesion. The cervical portion of the cord is most often affected by such lesions; consequently the segmental loss of pain and temperature usually involves the shoulders and arms, appearing in a so-called shawl distribution. The senses of touch, motion, position, and vibration are usually preserved until the lesion is large. This loss of pain and temperature perception with sparing of other sensory modalities is termed *dissociated* sensory loss. Loss of muscle stretch reflexes from damage to the anterior horn cells may occur in the distribution of the corresponding segments. Weakness, with atrophy and fasciculations because of involvement of lower motor neurons, is also detected in the distribution of the affected segments.

As intramedullary lesions progress, long tracts may be involved. Upper motor neuron signs below the level of the lesion result from involvement of the corticospinal tracts. Since the lateral spinothalamic tracts may be affected as the lesion extends laterally, loss of pain and temperature sensation develops below the level of the lesion on one or both sides, in addition to the segmental loss from damage to the crossing fibers. The sacral segments are occasionally spared because their representation in the spinothalamic tract is far lateral. Pain is less common with intramedullary lesions than with those in extramedullary sites.

Extramedullary cord lesions, either intradural or extradural, cause compression of the spinal cord and the nerve roots at the affected segment. The Brown-Sequard syndrome may result from lateral compression of the spinal cord. This syndrome, the result of damage to one-half the cord, consists of ipsilateral signs of dysfunction of the corticospinal tract and dorsal column below the level of the lesion, and contralateral reduction in pain and temperature perception below the level of the lesion. However, the syndrome is often incomplete; for example, ipsilateral motor deficits and contralateral loss of pain may appear without loss of motion, position, and vibratory sensations. The Brown-Sequard syndrome may also occur in some intramedullary lesions, such as multiple sclerosis (see Fig. 22D).

Compression of nerve roots by extramedullary lesions produces radicular pain and segmental motor and reflex changes (see p. 115). The location of radicular pain may be an important clue to the level of the lesion. Tenderness on pressure or percussion over the spinous process may be noted, particularly in extradural lesions affecting a vertebra.

Depending on the particular area of the cord involved, certain localizing features are distinctive. In the region of the foramen magnum and the high cervical area, combinations of spinal cord and brainstem signs may result. For example, lesions involving the spinal tract of the trigeminal nerve as it descends in the upper part of the cord may cause loss of pain and temperature sensation on the face. If the lesion is at the foramen magnum, the hypoglossal nerve may be affected.

Compression of the anterior spinal artery by a lesion in the region of the foramen magnum interferes with the blood supply to the cervical portion of the spinal cord, causing ischemia of the cord at levels lower than the lesion. The resulting dysfunction, for example in the hands (C8 through T1), therefore does not provide true localizing evidence of the motor and reflex changes.

Lesions in the cervical enlargement (C5 through T1) result in motor, sensory, and reflex signs in the arms and hands, as well as evidence of compression of the long ascending and descending tracts.

Lesions in the thoracic region cause radicular pain radiating around the rib cage anteriorly, which may be confused with pain from intrathoracic or intraabdominal disorders.

In the lumbosacral region, in addition to radicular signs and symptoms due to nerve root involvement, sphincter symptoms are of primary importance, as is pain in the region of the genitalia and anus. Involvement of the nerve roots by extramedullary tumors in this region may cause positive straight-leg-raising signs (see p. 115) and severe radicular pain.

THE CONUS MEDULLARIS AND CAUDA EQUINA

CONUS MEDULLARIS

The conus medullaris is small (less than 1 cm. in length) and is usually not affected without involvement of the adjacent roots. The important signs of damage to the conus medullaris include bilateral lower motor neuron loss affecting the legs, impairment of bladder and rectal sphincters, and sensory loss in the sacral dermatomes (saddle area). Tumors, trauma, and congenital malformations are the most frequent cause of disease in this region.

The muscles below the knees are usually affected by lesions of the conus medullaris, in particular the dorsiflexors, plantar flexors, invertors and evertors of the ankles, the long extensors of the toes, and the intrinsic foot muscles. Weakness is usually bilateral and has lower motor neuron characteristics—flaccidity, atrophy, and fasciculations. The Achilles reflex is usually lost bilaterally, but the quadriceps reflexes are preserved and may be brisk.

Sensory changes consist of decrease or loss of pain, temperature, and touch sensations in the perineum, the posterior thigh and leg, and the soles of the feet. When pain does occur, it is usually localized to these areas as well.

Urinary retention, overflow incontinence, and loss of sensation in the bladder also develop from lesions of the conus. Weakness of the anal sphincter with fecal incontinence occurs frequently, and impotence also is often associated with lesions of the conus.

CAUDA EQUINA

The cauda equina, consisting of anterior and posterior nerve roots from the caudal portion of the cord, is usually considered with the conus medullaris because of the anatomic association. The proximity of these structures to each other frequently results in damage to both, with a mixed clinical picture. As with the conus, tumors, trauma, and congenital malformations affect the cauda equina most frequently.

Disorders of the cauda equina are usually more painful than conus lesions because of the greater likelihood of irritation of posterior roots. Deficits are also more often spotty in distribution and may be confined to one lower extremity. As with conus medullaris lesions, flaccid paralysis of the leg muscles develops, but lesions of the cauda equina affect muscles above the knee as well as those below. Whatever the distribution of weakness, it is always of lower motor neuron type. Reflex alterations are asymmetrical; the Achilles and quadriceps reflexes are usually reduced or absent.

Sensory loss follows dermatomal distribution and is more profound in the peripheral aspect of the dermatomes. All dermatomes from the upper lumbar to the lower sacral may be involved. Bladder and rectal symptoms are similar to those developing with lesions of the conus medullaris. Pain and spasm on the straight-leg-raising test (see p. 115) is common and often noted bilaterally. There may be persistent low back pain, and often there is pain in the perineal and genital regions, with radiation down the legs.

TABLE 2. Symptoms and signs of common root lesions

Root	Location of Pain	Sensory Loss	Reflex Loss	Weakness & Atrophy
C5	Lower neck; tip of shoulder; arm	Deltoid area (inconsistent)	Biceps	Shoulder abductors; biceps
C6	Lower neck; medial scapula; arm; radial side of forearm	Radial side of hand; thumb; index finger	Biceps	Biceps
C7	Lower neck; medial scapula; precordium; arm; forearm	Index finger; middle finger	Triceps	Triceps
C8	Lower neck; medial arm & forearm; ulnar side of hand; 4th & 5th fingers	Ulnar side of hand; 4th & 5th fingers	. . .	Intrinsic hand muscles
L4	Low back; anterior & medial thigh	Anterior thigh	Quadriceps	Quadriceps
L5	Low back; lateral thigh; lateral leg; dorsum of foot; great toe	Great toe; medial side of dorsum of foot; lateral leg & thigh	. . .	Toe extensors; ankle dorsiflexors & evertors
S1	Low back; posterior thigh; posterior leg; lateral side of foot; heel	Lateral foot; heel; posterior leg	Achilles	Ankle dorsiflexion & plantar flexion

THE ANTERIOR AND POSTERIOR NERVE ROOTS

Although any of the anterior or posterior nerve roots on either side of the spinal cord can be involved in disease, most lesions involve one of the lower cervical (5 through 8), fifth lumbar, or first sacral roots. The most common root lesion is compression resulting from a herniated intervertebral disc, which in 95 percent of patients occurs at one of these sites. Other disorders affecting nerve roots include herpes zoster, trauma, and extramedullary tumors, such as meningioma, neurofibroma, and vertebral and paravertebral metastases.

Lesions of nerve roots usually lead to characteristic complaints, the most important being *radicular* pain, i.e., pain in the distribution of one of the dermatomal segments (Table 2; see also Fig. 24). The pain is often described as "shooting"; it radiates from the spine through the peripheral distribution of the root. It is aggravated by maneuvers which increase intraspinal pressure—coughing, sneezing, and straining—and also by movements of the spine and neck.

Pain is often the earliest clue in localizing the lesion. Later, motor, sensory, and reflex changes develop, which correspond to the root distribution suggested by the localization of the pain (Table 2). For example, if one of the muscle stretch reflexes is mediated by the affected root, the reflex will be diminished. Thus, involvement of the C7 root decreases or abolishes the triceps reflex; damage to the S1 nerve root results in loss of the Achilles reflex (see Fig. 25F). Because of the overlapping of dermatome distributions, objective sensory loss may be difficult to demonstrate if a lesion involves a single root. Such a loss is sometimes apparent, however, particularly in the C7 and S1 dermatome distributions. Within the dermatome the deficit is more marked in the periphery and usually consists of slight reduction of touch and pain perception.

Weakness is of lower motor neuron type. It may range from mild to very severe. For example, in the syndrome resulting from a C7 root lesion, reduction in triceps reflex, radicular pain, and slight sensory loss in the middle finger are more common than weakness of the muscles innervated by C7, which receive innervation from several other segments also. Thus, a part of the innervation of the muscles remains when this root is damaged. Tables 3 and 4 show the important patterns of segmental innervation.

One of the most valuable maneuvers in the analysis of root lesions is the straight-leg-raising test (SLR; Lasègue maneuver). The patient lies on his back, his legs extended. The examiner then lifts the patient's heel slowly, thus flexing the hip. If one or more of the posterior

TABLE 3. Segmental and peripheral innervation of muscles (upper extremity)

SPINAL CORD SEGMENTS

NERVE MUSCLES	Cervical				Thoracic
	5	6	7	8	1
Axillary					
Deltoid	■	■			
Musculocutaneous					
Biceps	■	■			
Brachialis	■	■			
Long Thoracic					
Serratus Anterior	■	■	■		
Suprascapular					
Supraspinatus	■	■			
Infraspinatus	■	■			
Radial					
Triceps		■	■	■	
Brachioradialis	■	■			
Ext Carpi Radialis L + B		■	■	■	
Supinator	■	■	■		
Extensor Digitorum		■	■	■	
Extensor Carpi Ulnaris			■	■	
Extensor Pollicis L + B			■	■	
Abductor Pollicis Longus			■	■	
Ulnar					
Flexor Carpi Ulnaris			■	■	■
Flexor Digit. Profundus*			■	■	■
Adductor Pollicis				■	■
Interossei				■	■
Flexor Pollicis Brevis - deep head				■	■
Lumbricals 3 and 4				■	■
Abductor Digiti Quinti				■	■
Opponens Digiti Quinti				■	■
Median					
Pronator Teres		■	■		
Flexor Carpi Radialis		■	■	■	
Flexor Digitorum Sublimis			■	■	■
Flexor Digitorum Profundus*			■	■	■
Abductor Pollicis Brevis				■	■
Opponens Pollicis				■	■
Flexor Pollicis Brevis				■	■
Lumbricals 1 and 2				■	■

*Innervated by more than one nerve.

roots contributing to the sciatic nerve is involved, this maneuver causes pain in the back and down the back of the thigh and leg, because of tension on the nerve. The test should be performed with each leg. Painful pulling sensations limited to the posterior knee area, not following the nerve root distribution, result from stretching of the hamstring muscles and have no clinical significance.

TABLE 4. Segmental and peripheral innervation of muscles (lower extremity)

SPINAL CORD SEGMENTS

NERVE / MUSCLES	Lumbar 1	2	3	4	5	Sacral 1	2	3
Obturator								
Adductor Longus and Brevis		▓	▓	▓				
Adductor Magnus*		▓	▓	▓				
Gracilis		▓	▓	▓				
Femoral								
Iliacus		▓	▓	▓				
Quadriceps		▓	▓	▓				
Sartorius		▓	▓	▓				
Sciatic								
Adductor Magnus*				▓	▓	▓		
Internal Hamstrings				▓	▓	▓	▓	
Biceps Femoris (Ext Hamstring)					▓	▓	▓	
Common Peroneal					▓	▓	▓	
Superficial Peroneal								
Peroneus Longus					▓	▓	▓	
Peroneus Brevis					▓	▓	▓	
Deep Peroneal								
Tibialis Anterior				▓	▓			
Extensor Digitorum Longus				▓	▓	▓		
Extensor Digitorum Brevis				▓	▓	▓		
Extensor Hallucis Longus				▓	▓	▓		
Tibial					▓	▓	▓	
Gastrocnemius-Soleus					▓	▓	▓	
Tibialis Posterior				▓	▓	▓		
Flexor Digitorum and Hallucis Longus					▓	▓	▓	
Inferior Gluteal Nerve					▓	▓	▓	
Gluteus Maximus					▓	▓	▓	
Superior Gluteal				▓	▓	▓		
Gluteus Medius and Minimus				▓	▓	▓		
Tensor Fasciae Lata				▓	▓	▓		

*Innervated by more than one nerve.

THE PLEXUSES

The cervical, brachial, and lumbosacral plexuses result from the rearrangement of the nerve roots in these areas. Because of this intermingling, lesions of the plexuses result in complex combinations of sensory and motor deficits. Lesions of the cervical plexus are uncommon and usually result from tumors, penetrating wounds, or violent injuries to the neck or shoulder. Brachial plexus lesions are more common and result from the same causes. The two main types, resulting from involvement of the upper and lower portions of the plexus, are discussed on page 76.

Damage to the lumbosacral plexus can result in various combinations of sensory and motor abnormalities in the lower extremities. In addition, bowel, bladder, and sexual functions may be impaired. Excepting war wounds, malignant tumors are the most common lesions affecting the lumbosacral plexus. The resulting pain and sensory and motor loss are difficult to distinguish from the clinical picture of lesions of the roots or peripheral nerves.

THE PERIPHERAL NERVES

Peripheral nerve lesions fall into three categories according to the nature of the damage and its extent in terms of the number of nerves involved. These are polyneuropathy (polyneuritis), mononeuritis multiplex, and mononeuropathy. Of these the one most frequently encountered is *polyneuropathy*, one of the neurologic manifestations of diabetes mellitus, malnutrition, heavy metal intoxication, and numerous other disorders. In typical form, this syndrome consists of symmetrical weakness and reduction of sensation in the distal portions of the extremities. The legs are invariably more affected than the arms regardless of cause; not uncommonly the arms are spared. In addition to these signs, produced by partial destruction of peripheral nerves, other complaints caused by irritation of nerve fibers are common. Included are an abnormal sensitivity of the skin when touched (dysesthesia), spontaneous unpleasant tingling and painful sensations (paresthesias), and tenderness of palpable peripheral nerves, and of muscles, particularly in the calf.

Weakness usually involves all distal muscles and ranges from mild to profound. It is symmetrical and most severe in the muscles of the calf and foot. Since weakness is of lower neuron type, atrophy occurs. Fasciculations are occasionally seen, although less commonly than in diseases of the anterior horn cells. Loss of muscle stretch reflexes is common, especially the Achilles reflex.

Trophic changes in the skin—thinness, dryness, and discoloration; superficial sores that heal poorly; and loss of hair—result from involvement of the autonomic fibers in the peripheral nerves. Edema and vasodilatation may also occur.

Mononeuritis multiplex denotes damage to "single nerves at multiple sites"—in other words, two or more of the peripheral nerves, not necessarily in the same extremity. This syndrome too is part of a wide variety of disorders including the collagen diseases, heavy metal poisoning, and diabetes mellitus.

The signs and symptoms of mononeuritis multiplex depend upon which of the major peripheral nerves are involved. The diagnosis depends on the examiner's knowledge of the sensory distribution and muscle innervation of these major nerves (see Tables 3 and 4; Fig. 22E).

More common than mononeuritis multiplex is the *single, isolated* peripheral nerve lesion—*mononeuropathy*—which commonly involves the peroneal, sciatic, femoral, ulnar, median, or radial nerve (Tables 3 and 4).

PERONEAL NERVE

This nerve is most vulnerable where it lies lateral to the fibula in the lateral aspect of the calf. Occasionally, pressure is exerted upon the nerve at this point by sitting with the legs crossed, by lying in bed with one leg over the other, particularly if the patient falls asleep, by prolonged pressure on the leg during anesthesia, or by a blow or a fall upon the leg. Recent weight loss may predispose to peroneal nerve injury—the decrease in subcutaneous tissue renders the nerve more susceptible to pressure.

The patient with a peroneal nerve lesion notes difficulty walking, in that he is unable to dorsiflex the ankle, thus catching or scraping the toes as he moves the foot forward (foot drop). Sensory complaints are uncommon, but occasionally a patient notes tingling on the dorsum of the foot and lateral calf. Examination reveals weakness of dorsiflexion and eversion of the ankle resulting from paresis of the anterior tibial and peroneal muscles. Sensory loss, if detectable, is confined to the lower lateral calf and dorsum of the foot (see Fig. 22E).

SCIATIC NERVE

The usual cause of sciatic mononeuropathy is chemical damage from injections of antibiotics or other substances into the nerve in its course in the buttock. Diabetes mellitus, trauma, neoplasm, and collagen disorders may also affect this nerve. The patient notes pain, tingling, and paresthesias along the back of the thigh and calf, and in the sole of the foot. In a complete sciatic nerve palsy, all the muscles below the knee are paralyzed. The patient walks with a slapping, foot-drop gait, as in peroneal nerve palsy. He can neither dorsiflex nor plantarflex the ankle. Sensory loss affects the back of the thigh, lateral and posterior calf, and the entire foot. The Achilles reflex is absent, but the quadriceps reflex is preserved.

FEMORAL NERVE

Diabetes mellitus is usually the cause of femoral neuropathy; trauma to the inguinal region, for example a bullet wound, is the only other common cause. The patient complains of difficulty walking and climbing stairs; the knee may buckle when bearing weight. Atrophy of the thigh may be apparent to the patient. Sensory complaints include numbness and pain on the anterior thigh and medial calf.

Examination reveals weakness of hip flexion and knee extension, atrophy of the quadriceps, reduced or absent quadriceps reflex, and sensory loss over the anterior thigh and medial calf.

ULNAR NERVE

This nerve is particularly susceptible to injury at the elbow, where it passes through the ulnar groove of the medial epicondyle of the humerus. Persons whose occupation requires that they rest their elbows on a desk for prolonged periods, for example, draftsmen, are particularly likely to develop compression mononeuropathy. Avoiding this position usually results in recovery. So-called *tardy ulnar palsy* may develop years after a fracture of the distal humerus.

Numbness and tingling usually initiate the disorder, but objective signs soon become obvious. The patient complains of numbness over the medial two fingers and medial side of the hand, then weakness of grip and difficulty using the fingers for fine movements. On examination, the sensory loss is usually easily demonstrable. Weakness of the interosseous muscles and the hypothenar muscles is present. In chronic cases a claw deformity of the fourth and fifth fingers may be noted. This includes flexion of the distal interphalangeal joints and hyperextension of the proximal joints.

In certain cases, transplantation of the nerve from the ulnar groove anteriorly at the elbow relieves compression and results in improvement.

MEDIAN NERVE

The median nerve is commonly damaged in two areas: the region of the elbow where it passes through the pronator teres muscles, and at the wrist in the carpal tunnel. In the former instance, the cause is usually trauma resulting from penetrating wounds, hypertrophy of the muscle, or carrying heavy objects which compress the tissues in the antecubital fossa. Median nerve injury in this area causes weakness and atrophy of the muscles in the forearm supplied by this nerve, and the thenar muscles, with resulting impairment of wrist and finger flexion and opposition of the thumb. Sensory loss is confined to the lateral side of the hand and the thumb, index, and middle fingers.

The *carpal tunnel syndrome* occurs more frequently in women than in men. It may be occupational, occurring in patients who hold their wrist in awkward positions of either forced extension or forced flexion for long periods—for example, the waitress who carries trays of dishes on the palm of her hand. The syndrome has been observed in association with diabetes, pregnancy, and hypothyroidism, as well as less common disorders. Sensory symptoms develop first. Typically, the patient awakens at night with tingling, numbness, and burning in her hands. In many cases the complaint involves the entire hand rather than typical median distribution. The patient gets up and shakes and massages her hands to gain relief. During the day, the symptoms are minor in the early stages, but become more persistent. An important point in the history is that the pain may involve the forearm in addition to the hand, thus suggesting a lesion of cervical roots or brachial plexus. After a variable period, motor complaints appear. The patient begins to have difficulty holding a pen or fork in the affected hand because of weakness of opposition of the thumb. Wasting of the thenar eminence may develop. The wrist and finger flexors are spared in lesions at the wrist, in contrast to more proximal lesions of the nerve. Cutting the transverse carpal ligament relieves the compression, and symptoms are usually relieved.

RADIAL NERVE

The radial nerve is most frequently damaged in the radial groove of the humerus. Fractures of the humerus, blows on the arm, and prolonged compression during heavy sleep or intoxication (Saturday night palsy) are common examples. The disorder is sometimes associated with diabetes mellitus, the collagen diseases, and lead poisoning.

Weakness of grip and inability to use the hand properly are the most common complaints. Normally a strong grip is associated with extension of the wrist. Although the finger flexors are innervated by the median and ulnar nerves, weakness of wrist extension and fixation reduces their mechanical advantage, with resulting weakness of grip. If the radial nerve is severely damaged a "wrist drop" occurs, in which extension of the wrist and fingers is absent. Sensory loss, if present, is confined to a small area just proximal to the thumb and index finger on the dorsum of the hand. If the injury is high in the upper arm, the triceps reflex may be reduced.

Other nerves occasionally damaged include the long thoracic, axillary, musculocutaneous, suprascapular, lateral femoral cutaneous, obturator, gluteal, and tibial (see Tables 3 and 4).

THE NEUROMUSCULAR JUNCTION

Myasthenia gravis is the most common disorder of the neuromuscular (myoneural) junction. It is characterized chiefly by weakness and ease of fatigue of skeletal muscles. Rare entities such as botulism and curare poisoning, however, also affect the junction, causing weakness or paralysis of skeletal muscle.

Normally, acetylcholine is released from nerve terminals at the neuromuscular junction. This neurotransmitter initiates depolarization of the muscle membrane, leading to contraction of the muscle fiber. The enzyme acetylcholinesterase controls and modifies the degree of stimulation by inactivating excess amounts of acetylcholine. Although the underlying cause of myasthenia gravis is not yet understood, it is clear that the effects are exerted primarily at the neuromuscular junction. A defect in the quantity, rate of release, or action of acetylcholine at this site results in inadequate muscle contraction.

The extraocular muscles are most frequently affected in myasthenia gravis, but weakness of the bulbar and extremity muscles is common. Ptosis and diplopia, often intermittent, are usually the initial complaints; dysarthria, dysphagia, neck weakness, and rapid fatigue and weakness of the arms and legs are also important features. Characteristically, weakness and fatigue worsen following day-long use of the affected muscles. The disease is occasionally life-threatening if the muscles of respiration are involved.

The distribution of the weakness is not of major help in diagnosis. Atrophy occurs in less than 5 percent of the cases; the reflexes are usually normal. Fasciculations do not occur. Because the weakness and fatigue appear without other clinical signs, the mistaken diagnosis of nonorganic weakness is occasionally made.

The diagnosis may be confirmed by injecting a substance which counteracts acetylcholinesterase (an anticholinesterase), thus potentiating acetylcholine and improving strength temporarily. Such substances include edrophonium (Tensilon) and neostigmine (Prostigmin).

THE MUSCLES

The most frequently encountered diseases of muscle are muscular dystrophy, polymyositis, and disorders associated with endocrine dysfunction, particularly hyperthyroidism. In children, muscular dystrophy is by far the most frequent and the most serious. Muscle diseases result in weakness, diminished or absent muscle stretch reflexes, and atrophy. Decreased reflexes and atrophy usually occur later than in diseases of the lower motor neuron, and fasciculations are absent.

The location of the weakness is helpful in distinguishing a muscle disease from a disease of the lower motor neuron. In the majority of instances, lower motor neuron disease (anterior horn cell or peripheral nerve) affects the distal muscles initially and remains most severe in this area, while primary muscle diseases usually affect the proximal (girdle) muscles initially. Exceptions to this rule occur, but are uncommon. When the differentiation of primary muscle from nerve disease cannot be ascertained from clinical examination, electromyography and muscle biopsy will often clarify the diagnosis.

The complaints mentioned most often by patients with muscle disease result from girdle weakness. The patient reports difficulty running, climbing stairs, and getting up from a sitting position, all functions of the hip girdle. Complaints referable to shoulder girdle weakness usually include weakness or fatigue of the arms in such activities as combing the hair or reaching up to high shelves. Children may offer no complaints, but their parents note clumsiness in their running and playing, and difficulty in getting up after having fallen. Sensory complaints are absent.

In an adult, the standard motor examination will suffice to demonstrate weakness of the girdle muscles. Special note should be made of the presence of atrophy and of tenderness of the muscles on palpation. In a child it may be difficult to test muscle strength. Proximal weakness in a child unable to cooperate in specific muscle testing may be evaluated by watching him rise from a supine position. If the pelvic muscles are weak, the child will "climb up himself," not jump up rapidly as does a normal child (Fig. 31). He will turn prone, then push his body from the floor with his arms. As his arms leave the floor, he quickly places his hands on his legs or thighs to aid in pushing the trunk upright.

Weakness of the shoulder girdle can be detected if the examiner places his hands under the patient's axillae and lifts the child. Normally a child's shoulder girdle muscles hold the arms strongly adducted so that he can be lifted. If the shoulder girdle musculature is weak, adduction is insufficient to support the child, the arms abduct as force is exerted, and the child slips downward through the physician's hands. "Winging" of the scapulae is another objective finding

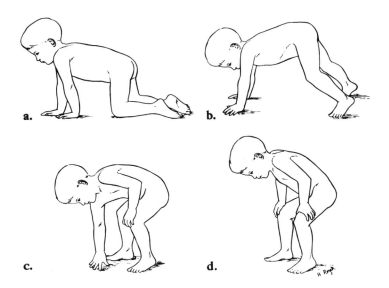

FIG. 31. Technique of rising used by a patient with weak hip and trunk muscles, e.g., muscular dystrophy (Gower's maneuver).

indicating weakness of those muscles normally holding the scapula tight against the thoracic cage.

The sensory examination is normal in patients with primary diseases of muscle.

In some instances, weakness occurs in muscles other than the girdles. Certain forms of muscular dystrophy cause weakness of neck, facial, and extraocular muscles. Similarly, polymyositis may involve neck and cranial musculature, sometimes seriously compromising functions of speech and swallowing.

Since muscular dystrophy is a hereditary disease, other members of the family may have similar complaints or present a similar appearance on examination.

Myotonia is detectable in some of the primary muscle diseases, notably myotonia congenita and myotonic dystrophy. Myotonia is defined as delayed relaxation of a muscle after normal contraction. It should not be confused with muscle tone as it is used elsewhere in relation to upper and lower motor neuron disease. To test for myotonia, ask the patient to grip an object firmly, then instruct him to quickly release his grip. When myotonia is present, his fingers will extend slowly and laboriously. Myotonia can also be detected by sharply percussing the muscle with a reflex hammer; again, a prompt contraction occurs followed by delayed relaxation. This is best observed in the thenar muscles and tongue muscles.

DIFFERENTIATION OF NERVE FROM MUSCLE DISEASE IN INFANCY

The syndrome of flaccid weak musculature in infancy—the "floppy infant"—is not rare. It may be caused by neural degeneration, primary muscle disease, endocrine derangement, and disorders of metabolism including "inborn errors" and defects of nutrition. Some of these causal disorders are hereditary. Some are rapidly fatal, while others progress very slowly or not at all.

Among the neurogenic disorders causing this syndrome are the relentlessly progressive *Werdnig-Hoffmann disease* and the relatively benign *Kugelberg-Welander syndrome*. In the first instance, muscle wasting is secondary to degeneration of anterior horn cells of the spinal cord, beginning in the first year of life and usually ending in death within a year. In the second instance there is proximal muscle atrophy resembling muscular dystrophy but with a neurogenic basis, and as no specific treatment is available, disability slowly advances.

The primary muscle disorders include congenital muscular dystrophy, benign congenital hypotonia, and rare disorders such as nemaline myopathy and central core disease, so named because of distinctive histologic features.

These infants exhibit diffuse weakness and hypotonicity; many have difficulty feeding, and cry weakly. Respirations are feeble. Reflexes may be elicited, but usually are weak or absent. Otherwise the neurologic examination is normal. The severity and distribution may be of weakness difficult to ascertain; therefore, laboratory aids such as electromyography and muscle biopsy are important in the diagnosis. In addition, ancillary studies including serum enzyme and other biochemical determinations are often necessary, as well as more recently developed histochemical and physiologic techniques which enable neurologists to detect finer points of distinction among disorders causing the "floppy infant" syndrome.

These disorders must also be differentiated from flaccidity secondary to spinal cord injuries (which in the infant cause hypotonia rather than spasticity), and congenital cerebral disorders of various types. Other causes of infantile hypotonia include mongolism (Down's syndrome), congenital heart disease, hypothyroidism (cretinism), and specific vitamin deficiencies (scurvy, rickets, etc.).

TESTS FOR MENINGEAL IRRITATION

The most important causes of meningeal irritation are bacterial, viral, and fungal infections and subarachnoid hemorrhage. Signs of meningeal irritation occasionally may occur during the course of some systemic illnesses (meningismus), but in such instances a lumbar puncture must be performed to exclude infectious meningitis.

Stiff neck (nuchal rigidity) is the most reliable sign of meningeal irritation, except during early infancy. Stiff neck is most easily detected by placing one hand under the occiput, when the patient is supine, and gently lifting the head. Resistance to this cervical flexion is easily perceived and is commonly accompanied by pain. Although highly suggestive of hemorrhage or meningitis, nuchal rigidity may develop in patients with increased intracranial pressure, particularly when the cause is a posterior fossa tumor.

The straight-leg-raising (Lasègue) sign of meningeal irritation is also performed with the patient supine. The thigh is flexed by the examiner, who lifts the leg from the heel, thus keeping the knee fully extended. A positive sign consists of limitation of hip flexion from either pain or involuntary resistance (hamstring muscle spasm), or both. In contrast to localized lumbosacral nerve root irritation (e.g., herniated intervertebral disc), which causes a unilateral Lasègue sign (p. 115), the sign is present bilaterally in the case of meningitis or subarachnoid hemorrhage. The basis for a positive Lasègue sign is stretching of the sciatic nerve, which in turn stretches inflamed or irritated nerve roots. Sudden passive dorsiflexion of the ankle while performing straight-leg-raising, therefore, may increase this stretch and result in increased pain and muscle resistance.

Kernig's sign is a classic maneuver but usually gives no more information than straight-leg-raising. The patient lies supine, with the hip and knee flexed. The knee is then passively extended. Knee extension is normally possible to an angle of about 135 degrees. Significant reduction in this angle, caused by pain and contraction of the hamstrings, is considered a positive test.

When these signs or other clinical features suggest meningeal irritation, lumbar puncture is necessary to determine whether the cause is infectious or hemorrhagic. Both conditions may produce severe headache and alteration of consciousness ranging from lethargy to coma; if these symptoms appear suddenly and develop very rapidly (within minutes) the cause is most likely a hemorrhage. If the meningitis is infectious, other signs of systematic infection, such as fever or skin rash, will suggest the diagnosis. Nevertheless, the cellular composition of the spinal fluid remains the most reliable diagnostic indicator.

CEREBROSPINAL FLUID

Examination of the cerebrospinal fluid (CSF) obtained by lumbar puncture aids in the diagnosis of several important neurologic disorders. However, unless the lumbar puncture is performed carefully and the fluid correctly analyzed, it has little or no value and may actually impede the diagnosis and management. Lumbar punctures are performed too frequently, often when there is little likelihood of obtaining useful information. The performance of this test tends to reassure the physician that he is not missing some obscure or puzzling neurologic problem. In most instances, however, there is clinical evidence for the existence of a neurologic problem, and an unexpected CSF abnormality leading to a diagnosis is a rare occurrence in the absence of neurologic signs and symptoms.

An important contraindication to lumbar puncture, therefore, is the lack of assurance that the results will be helpful. The presence of increased intracranial pressure or a known intracranial mass are other important contraindications unless hemorrhage or infection is to be excluded, because removal of additional fluid in the presence of increased intracranial pressure may cause a sudden shift in position (herniation) of one of the temporal lobes or of the cerebellar tonsils, with compression of vital brainstem centers. This has occasionally resulted in sudden death. Skin infection in the region of the puncture is an infrequent contraindication.

The principal indications for lumbar puncture are the need for confirmation of (1) *meningitis* and (2) *subarachnoid bleeding*. In addition, evaluation of the CSF pressure, serologic test for syphilis, and gamma globulin and protein determinations occasionally aid in diagnosis of other diseases.

TECHNIQUE OF LUMBAR PUNCTURE

The patient deserves an explanation of this procedure (as with any diagnostic procedure) before it is performed. He should be informed of its purpose and possible discomfort.

The most important step in the successful performance of a lumbar puncture is the positioning of the patient. He should lie on his side at the edge of the bed (not in the middle) or on an examining table. This will assure that he is lying on a horizontal rather than a sagging surface. A small pillow should be placed under the patient's head. His neck, hips, and knees are flexed so that he is, in effect, curled into a ball. He should not be straining or tense, however. Before proceeding, the examiner is wise to review the patient's position, adjusting the pillow and the degree of neck and hip flexion so that the spine is as perfectly horizontal as possible.

The skin is prepared with an antiseptic solution. Since many of these solutions contain iodine, the patient should be asked if he has ever had skin reactions to iodine solutions, and if so, a substitute is used. In any case, it is advisable to remove the iodine from the skin with alcohol. The physician then puts on sterile gloves and covers the lumbar area with a standard sterile drape which has a 6-inch opening in the center.

Lumbar puncture is usually performed in the vertebral interspace between L4 and L5 or L5 and S1. The L4–L5 interspace is directly opposite the iliac crest; with the drape in place the crest can be palpated and the interspace located. This interspace and those adjacent are palpated so that the one with the widest opening may be chosen. Lumbar puncture should not be done above the L3–L4 interspace because of the danger of penetrating the conus medullaris.

The skin overlying the interspace is infiltrated with approximately 0.5 ml. of procaine hydrochloride, or a similar local anesthetic agent. It is not necessary to infiltrate deeper structures.

The physician is now ready to perform the puncture. A 20-gauge lumbar puncture needle is the best choice, but if a myelogram or Queckenstedt test (see below) is to be performed, an 18-gauge needle is used. The needle is introduced in the midline in a perfectly horizontal plane, the point directed approximately 15 to 20 degrees rostrally. At a depth of 1½ to 2½ inches (approximately) a sudden yield is perceived as the needle advances. The stylet is then withdrawn to detect fluid appearing at the end of the needle. If none appears, the needle may be rotated 180 degrees in one direction or the other—this may initiate or improve the flow. Cautious advancement of the needle another few millimeters may also improve flow. Occasionally, a nerve root may be touched by the point of the needle, causing the patient to complain of pain in the leg or perineal area. Rotation or slight withdrawal of the needle alleviates this problem.

The bevel of the needle must be entirely within the subarachnoid space to ensure satisfactory measurement of pressure and sampling of fluid. To test adequacy of needle placement, ask the patient to cough, or have an assistant compress the patient's abdomen. The resulting increase in intraabdominal pressure is transmitted to the subarachnoid space via the spinal veins, causing a rise in CSF pressure; failure of the pressure to rise with this maneuver indicates a need to adjust the needle by rotation or advancement.

After the needle has entered the subarachnoid space, the patient should be reassured that the major portion of the procedure is over and that he will feel no more discomfort. He may extend his neck and legs carefully to make his position more comfortable. He should take a few deep breaths and relax as much as possible.

The CSF pressure is first measured. A three-way stopcock with manometer is attached to the needle and the fluid allowed to rise in the manometer. Initially high CSF pressure often returns to normal during a 2- or 3-minute wait which allows the patient to relax. No pressure should be assumed abnormal unless all these steps are taken.

If the CSF pressure is above 200 mm. and the examiner is convinced that the patient is adequately relaxed, then only the CSF remaining in the manometer should be drained into a tube for analysis. However, if meningitis is a consideration, enough fluid should be cautiously removed to ensure an adequate sample for complete bacteriologic evaluations. The needle is then removed.

If the pressure is normal, samples are then collected in three tubes, the first tube containing 1 to 2 ml., the second approximately 10 ml., and the third 1 to 2 ml. Additional fluid may be required in special instances such as cytologic evaluation.

In suspected mass lesions (e.g., tumors) of the spinal cord, the *Queckenstedt test* may yield important information. An assistant is required. After establishing the base-line CSF pressure reading, the assistant compresses both internal jugular veins for 10 seconds while the examiner observes the manometer. Normally, the CSF pressure should rise promptly to at least double its base-line value; in many cases, it rises much higher. (Coughing or abdominal compression does not give equivalent information.)

After compression for 10 seconds, the pressure on the internal jugular veins is released quickly. The CSF pressure should promptly fall to base-line or nearly base-line levels. Failure of the normal rise is most often due to faulty positioning of the needle or inadequate compression of the jugular veins. Failure of the expected rise apart from artifacts, however, indicates obstruction of the spinal subarachnoid space. This block may be caused by a tumor, a herniated intervertebral disc, an epidural hemorrhage or abscess, or cervical spondylosis.

If the Queckenstedt test is positive, 3 to 6 ml. of iodophendylate (Pantopaque) should be introduced through the needle for immediate myelography. *The Queckenstedt test should never be performed if any intracranial lesion is suspected, because of the danger of herniation.*

If the contraindications are observed, lumbar puncture is very rarely attended by complication, with the exception of a characteristic headache. This headache occurs in a distinct minority of patients; it seems to be more frequent in people with preexisting knowledge of its occurrence. Typically, the headache is produced by or accentuated by the upright position and promptly relieved by recumbency. The condition is temporary, seldom lasting more than a day or two.

ANALYSIS OF THE CEREBROSPINAL FLUID

Before analyzing the CSF, the physician must be certain of his objective. Too commonly, a crucial lumbar puncture is performed only to be wasted because the ensuing analysis is incomplete or carelessly performed.

The first step is to inspect the fluid. Normally, it is clear and colorless, indistinguishable from water, with which it can be compared. If it appears pink or bloody, the differentiation between puncture trauma and subarachnoid hemorrhage from a pathologic process must be made immediately. If the fluid clears as more is removed, the tap was probably traumatic. Next, a small amount of the CSF is centrifuged and the supernatant inspected. If the supernatant is xanthochromic, subarachnoid hemorrhage from a preexisting condition has occurred; if it is clear, the blood came from either needle trauma or very recent subarachnoid hemorrhage. Finally, the red blood cell count in the first tube is compared with that of the third: the two counts should be approximately the same if there is a preexisting subarachnoid hemorrhage; but in a traumatic tap, many more red blood cells are present in the first tube than in the third.

The next procedure is a complete cell count. Undiluted CSF is flooded into a standard hematology counting chamber. All nine squares should be counted and the results multiplied by 10/9 to give the total number of cells per cubic millimeter. The procedure is then repeated, using a pipette previously rinsed with glacial acetic acid to lyse red cells. The white cell count is thus obtained, and the difference is the red cell count. If there are more than 5 white cells per cubic millimeter, a differential count should be obtained by centrifuging a sample of fluid, making a film, and staining it with Wright's stain. A differential count cannot be made accurately on unstained spinal fluid in the counting chamber.

Table 5 indicates the cerebrospinal fluid abnormalities in various diseases.

If the white blood cell count is abnormal or if an infection is suspected, a sterile sample of CSF must be sent to the bacteriology laboratory for appropriate cultures. If an infection was suspected before the lumbar puncture, it is wise to collect a few drops of CSF directly into a culture tube containing broth for immediate incubation. Send all specimens for bacteriologic cultures to the laboratory immediately; delay decreases the chance of a positive culture.

Appropriate bacteriologic stains of dried smears of CSF should be prepared in all cases of suspected infections. An India ink preparation should be obtained in any case where cryptococcosis is a possibility. These budding organisms may also be seen in Wright-stained smears of good quality.

Another sample of fluid should be sent to the laboratory for protein, gamma globulin, and glucose determinations, as well as the serologic test for syphilis—1 or 2 ml. of CSF is all that is required except in cases where more refined tests for syphilis are indicated. A quick but very rough estimate of CSF protein level can be obtained from the *Pandy test*. One drop of CSF is added to 1 ml. of saturated phenol (Pandy reagent). Formation of a white precipitate indicates a protein level above 50 mg. per 100 ml.

Protein in CSF is normally less than 45 mg. per 100 ml. Many pathologic states are associated with high CSF protein, and therefore no specific diagnosis can be made from this finding. The highest values usually indicate spinal cord tumors, either primary or metastatic, especially when the Queckenstedt test is positive. Other conditions causing very high values are the Guillain-Barré syndrome, subarachnoid hemorrhage, and bacterial and fungal meningitis.

TABLE 5. Cerebrospinal fluid abnormalities

Disease	Pressure	Cell Type: Approx. Counts	Protein	Sugar	Other
Acute purulent meningitis	Increased	Polymorph., 100 to several thousand	Elevated—to 1,000 mg.	Reduced to absent	Organisms may be seen on gram stain
Tuberculous meningitis	Increased	Lymphocytes, 50 to 500	Elevated—to 1,000 mg.	Reduced	Organisms may be seen on Ziehl-Nielsen stain
Cryptococcus meningitis	Increased	Lymphocytes, 10 to 500	Elevated	Reduced	Organisms seen on india ink or Wright-stained preparations
Meningeal malignancy: carcinoma, melanoma, leukemia	Normal to increased	Lymphocytes, 10 to 500	Elevated	Normal to reduced	Malignant cells identified on cytologic examination
Viral meningitis	Normal to increased	Lymphocytes, 10 to 300	Normal to elevated	Normal	
General paresis	Normal	Lymphocytes, 10 to 300	Normal to elevated	Normal	Strongly positive serologic tests; elevated gamma globulin

Tabes dorsalis	Normal	Lymphocytes, 10 to 300 (none in late cases)	Normal to elevated	Normal	Positive serologic tests; elevated gamma globulin (may be normal in late cases)
Brain abscess	Elevated	Polymorph. or lymphocytes, normal to thousands	Normal to elevated	Normal	
Multiple sclerosis	Normal	Occasional lymphocytes, usually very few	Usually normal	Normal	Frequently elevated gamma globulin
Guillain-Barré syndrome	Usually normal	Usually normal; occasionally a few lymphocytes	Normal early; to 1,000 mg./100 ml. later	Normal	
Cerebral thrombosis	Usually normal	Polymorph. or lymphocytes, usually very few; occasionally up to 50 polymorph. or lymphocytes	Normal to 100	Normal	
Brain tumors	Normal to high	Mostly lymphocytes, normal to 100	Variable: high in acoustic neuroma	Normal	
Subarachnoid hemorrhage	Normal to high	Many RBC, grossly bloody; xanthochromic supernatant	High	Normal	

Gamma globulin content is normally less than 10% of the total protein. Values above 14% of the total protein strongly suggest multiple sclerosis or syphilis.

Cerebrospinal fluid glucose is markedly reduced in bacterial meningitis and tuberculous meningitis but is normal in virus infections. Normally, the CSF glucose content is two-thirds of the blood glucose, which *must* be determined simultaneously.

When a malignancy is suspected, a sample of fluid may be examined for the presence of malignant cells. Five to 10 ml. of fluid is adequate, since there is little chance of finding abnormal cells by examining larger amounts.

Plain x-ray films should be obtained before more complex examinations such as arteriography, air encephalography, or myelography are performed. While plain films are often normal despite the presence of neurologic lesions, they sometimes yield important diagnostic information.

Several abnormalities can be detected on plain films of the skull; Figure 32 shows some examples of normal and abnormal skull films.

1. Abnormal size and contour of the cranium resulting from congenital malformations or mass lesions—for example, hydrocephalus, microcephaly, craniosynostosis
2. Fractures
3. Abnormal lucencies: Destruction or erosion of bone by tumors or other means
4. Abnormal densities: Meningiomas and certain other tumors may result in an osteoblastic reaction of the skull
5. Alterations in the sella turcica: The commonest are enlargement resulting from pituitary tumors and erosion of the floor of the sella, particularly along the anteroinferior margin of the dorsum sellae, as a result of generalized increase in intracranial pressure
6. Enlargement of the foramina of exit of the cranial nerves due to neoplasms: Most frequent are acoustic neuromas, which produce enlargement of the internal acoustic meatus, and optic nerve glioma, which expands the optic foramen
7. Displacement of the pineal gland: This structure is normally calcified in 50 to 60% of adults; a mass lesion will displace the pineal gland to the opposite side, an atrophic lesion, to the same side (less than 3 mm. deviation is not conclusive)
8. Abnormal calcifications: Calcification may occur within a tumor, usually those that are growing slowly; abnormal intracranial calcification also occurs in tuberculomas and disorders such as Sturge-Weber syndrome, tuberous sclerosis, toxoplasmosis, and cytomegalic inclusion body disease; despite the rarity of these diseases, the radiographic appearance may be of major diagnostic significance
9. Abnormalities of the paranasal sinuses that relate to neurologic problems: For example, sinus infection might be related to a brain abscess or meningitis
10. Relation of skull to cervical vertebrae: The upper portion of

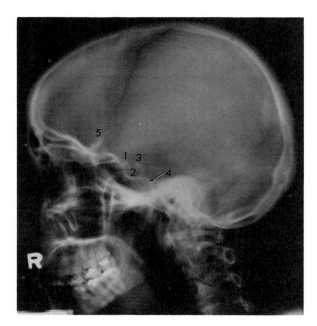

A

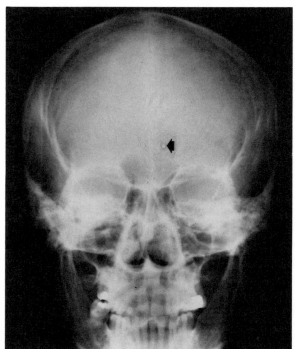

B

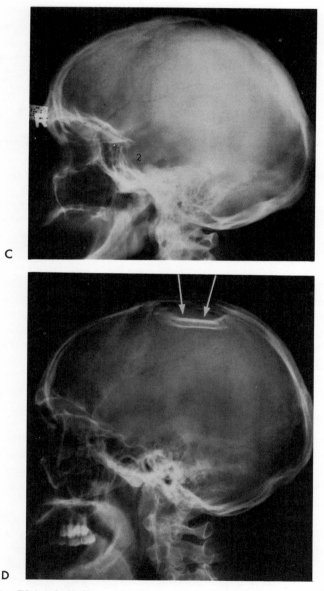

C

D

FIG. 32. Plain skull films. (A) Normal lateral skull film. *1*, anterior clinoid processes; *2*, sella turcica; *3*, posterior clinoid processes; *4*, clivus; *5*, greater wings of sphenoids. (B) Posteroanterior skull film. The calcified pineal gland (*arrow*) is shifted from the midline to the left due to a right hemisphere tumor. (C) Pituitary adenoma. Compare size of sella turcica (*2*) to that in A. (D) Depressed skull fracture (*arrows*).

the cervical spine is seen on plain skull films; congenital abnormalities of the relation of the skull to the vertebrae may result in neurologic symptoms; these abnormalities result in distortion and compression of the brainstem and upper cervical cord

Because of the variety of pathologic lesions visualized on plain spine films, they should be obtained in every patient with a neurologic picture suggesting a spinal cord or nerve root disorder. They are particularly important in patients with a history of trauma, suspected tumors, arthritis, and herniated intervertebral discs.

Fractures of the vertebrae are usually detected by routine spine x-rays. Pathologic fractures, those secondary to neoplasm in the bone, are also visible. Intramedullary tumors of the spinal cord may produce no changes on plain films, but as they enlarge, the size of the spinal canal may increase. Tumors may erode the pedicles. Neurofibromas may result in enlargement of the intervertebral foramina. Metastatic tumors of the vertebrae may result in osteoblastic or osteolytic changes in the vertebrae. The changes of osteoarthritis and rheumatoid arthritis of the spine are often seen on plain films. The intervertebral space may be narrowed if the disc at that interspace has herniated.

Tuberculosis, spina bifida, fusion of vertebrae, metabolic bone disorders, abnormalities of calcium metabolism, and abnormal curvatures of the spine are examples of disorders associated with characteristic abnormalities visible on routine spine films.

CEREBRAL ANGIOGRAPHY

In cerebral angiography, the blood vessels of the brain are visualized by means of serial radiographic films taken in various planes following injection of a contrast substance into the arterial (occasionally venous) circulation. The contrast substance is a radiopaque organic iodine compound which is soluble in water.

The site of injection depends on which part of the cerebral circulation is in question, and this in turn depends on the patient's history and physical signs. Formerly, the techniques involved surgical exposure of the common carotid artery followed by injection of the contrast substance, but percutaneous injection with a special needle is now the standard procedure. The same technique may be applied to the vertebral artery, to visualize the circulation of the brainstem and cerebellum, but this procedure is more difficult and has largely been abandoned.

Another technique that has been used is retrograde brachial angiography. Here the contrast substance is injected against the flow of arterial blood, which must be overcome by the pressure of the injection. As the contrast medium reaches the origin of the vertebral artery on the side of injection, some of it enters this vessel. With right brachial injection, some of the contrast medium enters the carotid system. On the left, the substance enters the descending aorta rather than the carotid artery.

The most satisfactory technique for cerebral angiography (but only in experienced hands) involves catheterization of the femoral artery. A specially shaped catheter is passed through the artery into the descending aorta, up to the arch of the aorta, and with careful fluoroscopic control, its tip is placed in the desired vessel or vessels. Because the entire extracranial and intracranial cerebral circulation can thus be studied, femoral artery catheterization is replacing such techniques as retrograde brachial angiography, which requires multiple arterial punctures to fully evaluate cerebral circulation and usually gives an examination of poorer diagnostic quality.

Cerebral angiography can give information of great value. It is the best method for studying disease of the blood vessels themselves, such as atherosclerosis, where there is narrowing of the vessels and consequent impairment of circulation. Aneurysms of cerebral blood vessels are usually demonstrable by angiography. Congenital malformations of the blood vessels are also best demonstrated by angiography.

When collections of blood above or beneath the dura mater (epidural or subdural hematoma) are present, angiography of the appropriate blood vessels reveals any displacement or shift of the adjacent vessels on the surface of the brain and also those along the midline of the brain toward the opposite side.

Similarly, mass lesions within the brain itself are indirectly demonstrated by angiography because of displacement of the adjacent blood vessels, either arteries or veins, from their normal position. Primary and metastatic brain tumors, cerebral abscesses, localized cerebral hemorrhages, and cysts are all demonstrable by this method. Tumors often contain abnormal blood vessels of characteristic appearance; a tumor "stain" is sometimes seen.

Dilation of the ventricular system from obstruction in the flow of cerebrospinal fluid can be detected by the displacement of blood vessels surrounding the ventricles. Several characteristic lesions detected by angiography are included in Figure 33.

Numerous complications of angiography have been reported, but with careful attention to detail and good judgment regarding the choice of the technique, adverse reactions are unlikely. Damage to the carotid artery sometimes occurs when some of the contrast substance is inadvertently injected into the vessel wall, leading to occlu-

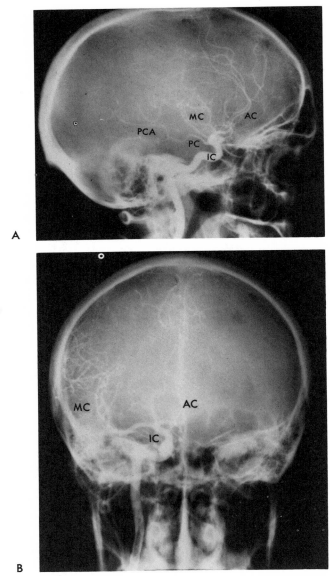

FIG. 33. Arteriography. (A) Normal lateral carotid arteriogram. (*AC* = anterior cerebral artery; *MC* = middle cerebral artery; *IC* = internal carotid artery; *PC* = posterior communicating artery; *PCA* = posterior cerebral artery. (B) Normal anteroposterior carotid arteriogram.

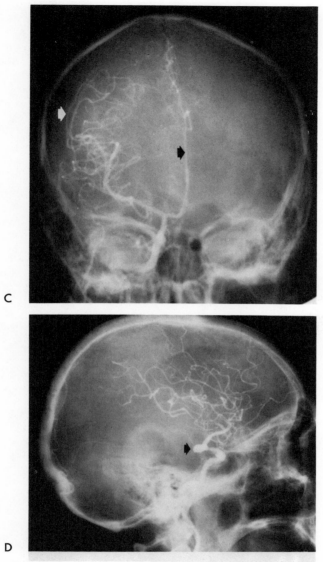

(C) Right subdural hematoma. *Arrows* indicate extent of subdural blood and shift of anterior cerebral artery toward the left. (D) Aneurysm (*arrow*) of posterior communicating artery.

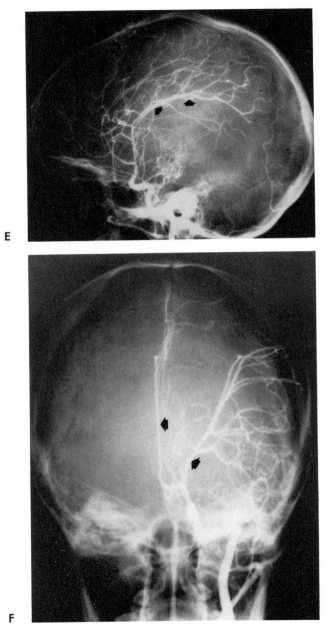

E

F

FIG. 33 (*Continued*). (E) Left temporal lobe tumor, lateral view. Note marked elevation of middle cerebral artery (*arrows*). Compare with A. (F) Left temporal lobe tumor, frontal view. Note shift of anterior cerebral vessels toward the right and medial and upward displacement of middle cerebral vessels (*arrows*).

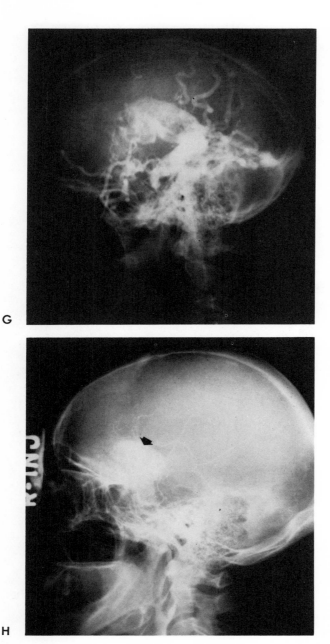

(G) Congenital arteriovenous malformation. Note huge tangle of abnormal blood vessels. (H) Meningioma of sphenoid wing, showing tumor "stain" (*arrow*).

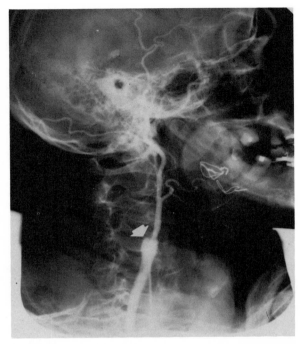

FIG. 33 *(Continued)*. (I) Complete occlusion of internal carotid artery *(arrow)*. External carotid artery fills well.

sion of the vessel. This may result in hemiparesis and other focal neurologic deficits. With increasing use of femoral catheter techniques, this is now a rarity. Spasm of the arterial system has occurred in some cases, presumably because of irritation from the needle or the contrast substance; this also may result in hemiparesis. A hematoma may form because of leakage and collection of blood around the site of injection, particularly when several punctures have been made or postoperative care is inadequate. Serious allergic reactions to the contrast substance have occurred only in rare instances.

AIR ENCEPHALOGRAPHY

Air encephalography is a radiologic technique in which air is introduced either into the lumbar subarachnoid space (pneumoencephalography), from which it passes into the ventricular system, or directly into the ventricular system (ventriculography). The air serves as a contrast substance. Radiographic films are then made with the head in various positions in order to visualize all of the ventricular system and those portions of the subarachnoid space that are of particular interest. Either technique is of value in determining size, relationships, and contours of the ventricular system. Pneumoencephalography may also aid in detecting atrophy of the cerebral cortex and mass lesions encroaching on the subarachnoid space, particularly in the sellar region.

Air contrast techniques, while formerly of great importance, are now less commonly utilized for detection of brain tumors, especially in the hemispheres, as angiographic techniques are becoming more sophisticated and accurate, as well as entailing less risk and discomfort.

Pneumoencephalography is usually contraindicated for patients with signs of increased intracranial pressure, because of the danger of herniation of one or both temporal lobes through the tentorium, with midbrain compression, when the CSF pressure is abruptly lowered through the lumbar puncture needle (see "Technique of Lumbar Puncture"). Ventriculography is performed in such cases, because reduction of pressure above rigid intracranial structures such as the tentorium entails less risk.

PNEUMOENCEPHALOGRAPHY

Pneumoencephalography is performed by injecting air through a needle into the spinal subarachnoid space after lumbar puncture. Small increments of 5 to 10 ml. of air or oxygen are introduced while a smaller amount of fluid is usually removed. When the patient is in a sitting position, the air rises and enters the ventricular system and intracranial subarachnoid spaces. By proper positioning of the head, air can be introduced into the various portions of the ventricular system and subarachnoid cisterns as deemed necessary from the suspected nature and location of the lesion.

Pneumoencephalography is of particular value in searching for tumors adjacent to the ventricular system or in the pituitary region, unless the procedure is contraindicated by increased intracranial pressure. It is also valuable in the study of congenital malformations of the brain, especially those which cause alterations in the ventricular system, such as adjacent cysts. The presence of focal cerebral or cerebellar cortical atrophy can usually be detected by pneumoencephalography. Dilatation of the ventricles resulting from generalized brain atrophy (hydrocephalus ex vacuo) is easily demonstrated. Figure 34 illustrates normal and several abnormal pneumoencephalograms.

Pneumoencephalography produces headache in most patients, occasionally severe and accompanied by signs of meningeal irritation, including stiff neck and the presence of inflammatory cells in the spinal fluid. With bedrest, high fluid intake, analgesics, and sedatives, these symptoms usually disappear in a day or two.

VENTRICULOGRAPHY

Ventriculography entails the introduction of air (or occasionally a radiopaque substance) through a needle which is passed through the brain substance into one of the lateral ventricles, following placement of a burr hole in the skull. The ventricular system is well visualized by this technique, but the subarachnoid space is not.

The indications for ventriculography have decreased in recent years primarily because of improved quality and versatility of cerebral angiography.

Ventriculography is of particular value in the study of lesions which cause hydrocephalus by obstructing CSF in its normal flow from the lateral ventricles into the third ventricle, the aqueduct of Sylvius, and the fourth ventricle. Congenital obstruction of the aqueduct, tumors in the posterior fossa of the skull obstructing the fourth ventricle, and tumors within the third ventricle can be demonstrated. Lesions obstructing the aqueduct or fourth ventricle are seen to particular advantage using a radiopaque substance such as iodophendylate, because it has greater contrast than air. Figure 35 illustrates a ventriculogram from a patient with hydrocephalus.

Because it involves a direct approach through the brain, the procedure entails risks, the most important of which is hemorrhage from a blood vessel accidentally injured by the needle.

MYELOGRAPHY

Myelography is a radiologic diagnostic technique in which a radio-opaque contrast substance is introduced into the subarachnoid space via lumbar puncture. The procedure is carried out under fluoroscopic control. By tilting the patient up and down on a special table, the entire extent of the spinal subarachnoid space can be outlined. The contrast substance can be brought to the cervicomedullary junction and into the posterior cranial fossa in cases where mass lesions in this area are suspected.

Myelography is most often performed to aid in the diagnosis of herniated intervertebral discs in either the lumbar or cervical regions. The test is also of great value in the diagnosis of tumors encroaching on the spinal subarachnoid space. Intramedullary tumors usually cause a diffuse, rather symmetrical widening of the spinal cord which is demonstrable by myelography. Syringomyelia, hydromyelia, and intramedullary hemorrhage have a similar appearance. Tumors lying within the subarachnoid space, such as neurofibromas and meningiomas, have a characteristic myelographic appearance; usually they are sharply outlined by the contrast substance. Tumors outside the subarachnoid space, for example a metastatic tumor involving a vertebra, indent the dura and produce a less sharply outlined, irregular shadow.

Arteriovenous malformations on the surface of the spinal cord or in the subarachnoid space may be demonstrated by myelography. These are uncommon lesions sometimes confused with tumors and degenerative diseases.

Arachnoiditis, a chronic proliferative inflammation of arachnoidal tissue causing distortion and compression of the cord and nerve roots, may also be detected. This condition, like arteriovenous malformation, is often confusing and difficult to distinguish from tumors and degenerative processes.

Traumatic lesions of the vertebrae and of the spinal cord can sometimes be identified by this technique if the clinical picture is unclear, but the decision for myelography must be carefully weighed, since the procedure may complicate the injury. It is performed only when the localization of the lesion is essential to surgical intervention.

Figure 36 illustrates some of the common abnormalities demonstrable by myelography.

Myelography is accomplished by means of a standard lumbar punc-

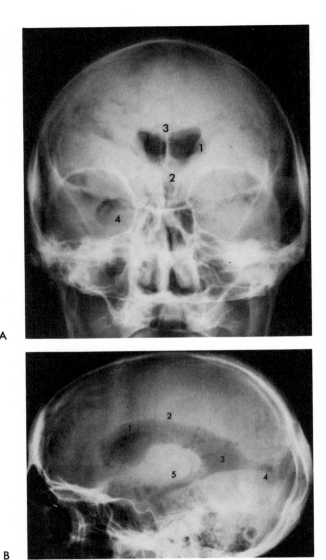

A

B

FIG. 34. Pneumoencephalography. (A) Normal frontal view. *1*, lateral ventricle (body and anterior horn); *2*, third ventricle; *3*, septum pellucidum; *4*, right temporal horn. (B) Normal lateral view. The lateral ventricles are well filled but the third and fourth ventricles are not. *1*, anterior horn; *2*, body; *3*, trigone; *4*, occipital horn; *5*, temporal horn. (C) Normal fourth ventricle and posterior third ventricle. *1*, suprapineal recess; *2*, posterior third ventricle; *3*, massa intermedia; *4*, aqueduct of Sylvius; *5*, fourth ventricle. (D) Diffuse atrophy of the right cerebral hemisphere. Note dilated right lateral ventricle (posterior aspect is visualized) as well as asymmetrical cranial vault with reduced capacity and thicker wall on the right (*arrows*).

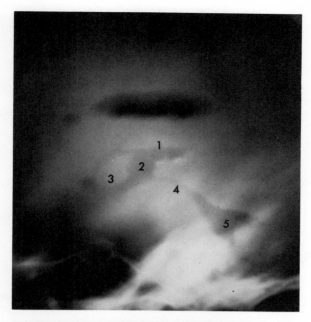

C

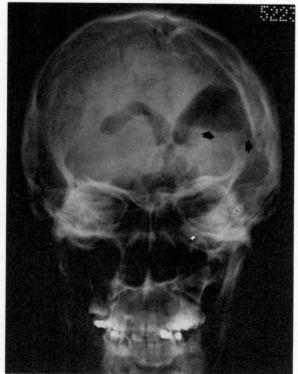

D

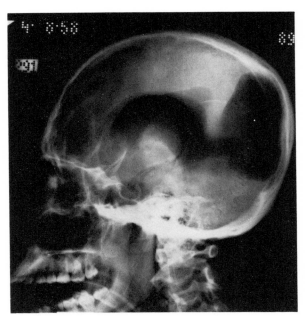

A

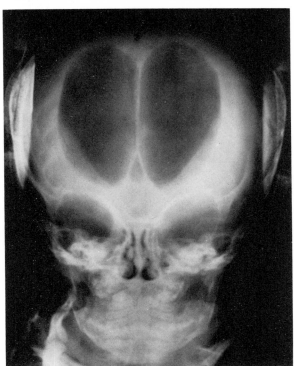

B

152

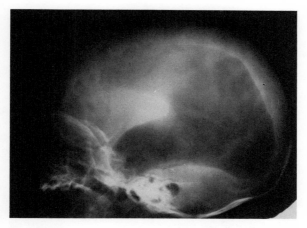

C

FIG. 35. Ventriculography. (A) Ventriculogram showing large cyst communicating with lateral ventricle. (B, C) Ventriculograms showing congenital hydrocephalus.

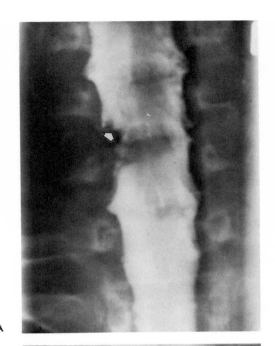

A

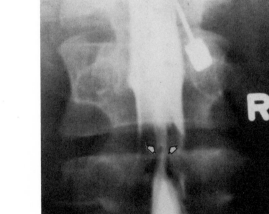

B

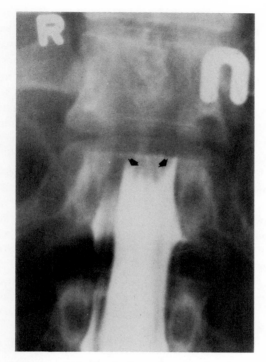

C

FIG. 36. Myelography. (A) Cervical myelogram showing herniated cervical disc (*arrow*). (B) Lumbar myelogram showing large herniated lumbar disc (*arrows*). (C) Thoracic myelogram. The contrast column is interrupted by a meningioma (*arrows*).

ture. The contrast substance is introduced through the needle with a syringe. After a small amount has been introduced, the site is viewed through the fluoroscope to ensure that the contrast substance has entered the subarachnoid space and not the subdural space. The injection then continues with 6 to 15 ml. of contrast medium, the larger amounts being used when the cervical region is of special interest. The patient is then tilted upward in order to fill the caudal sac of the subarachnoid space while it is inspected under the fluoroscope. The patient is then slowly tilted downward and the contrast substance is observed as it flows toward the cervical region. The tilting is carefully controlled so that it can be interrupted for closer inspection. As the contrast substance advances through the thoracic region, the patient's head is hyperextended to prevent the substance from flowing into the posterior fossa of the skull. In suspected posterior fossa masses the contrast substance is allowed to enter the posterior fossa to outline this region—posterior fossa cisternography. Standard films are made in various positions as the procedure is carried out.

After a complete survey of the spinal canal, the contrast substance is pooled in the region of the needle and as much as possible is removed by aspiration under fluoroscopic control. Any contrast substance remaining is gradually absorbed.

Myelography has a fairly high incidence of morbidity but not of a serious nature. Many patients complain of backache because the large-gauge needle has been in place for periods sometimes exceeding an hour. The discomfort usually ceases in a few days. The likelihood of headache is increased in this procedure above that in routine lumbar puncture. Occasionally, there is a mild meningeal inflammation, producing headache and stiff neck, which lasts for a few days.

Since the contrast medium used for myelography contains iodine, thyroid function tests which involve measurement of iodine may be altered. Therefore, any indicated thyroid studies should be performed before myelography whenever possible.

ISOTOPE ENCEPHALOGRAPHY (BRAIN SCAN)

Brain scanning is an important technique for the demonstration of brain tumors, brain abscess, and subdural hematoma. It may also be helpful in evaluating cerebral infarction, arteriovenous malformation, and intracerebral hemorrhage.

Several isotopes have been used for brain scans, including radioiodinated serum albumin (RISA), mercury 203, mercury 197, and most recently technetium 99m. The latter isotope is more satisfactory than some of the others because of its very short half-life (6 hours) and the minimal danger of radiation exposure.

The procedure is carried out after intravenous or intramuscular administration of the radioisotope; after a suitable delay, regional variations in intensity of emitted radiation are recorded by means of a moving scintillation scanner. Under certain conditions the radio-isotope accumulates in an area of abnormality in greater amounts than in normal tissue, thus providing a contrast when the entire brain is scanned. The reason for the accumulation of radioisotopes in areas of disease is not known. It may be related to the degree of vascularity of the lesion or to regional changes in the blood-brain barrier.

Scans are much more likely to be abnormal in the presence of highly malignant tumors, such as glioblastoma multiforme and metastases; slower-growing tumors usually show less uptake (Fig. 37). In cerebro-vascular occlusion with brain infarction, the scan frequently becomes positive during the first two or three weeks after the occlusion, when there is acute tissue damage and repair, but usually returns to normal after several weeks. Scans are usually positive in patients with brain abscesses and large subdural hematomas.

Unless deemed essential, brain scans are avoided in children and during early pregnancy because of the potentially harmful effects of radiation—minimal with technetium, however. Otherwise, the pro-cedure is safe and free from discomfort, except that it requires the patient to remain still during the scanning period, which lasts from one-half to one hour. This is difficult to achieve with some patients, and sedation may be required.

ELECTROMYOGRAPHY AND NERVE CONDUCTION STUDIES

Clinical electromyography is a technique for studying the electric potentials produced by striated muscles. The potentials are recorded by the insertion of needle electrodes into muscles, amplified, and trans-mitted to an oscilloscope, where they are displayed on the screen; they may be made audible, after amplification, by a loudspeaker. The test is especially valuable for the study of muscle weakness because it often differentiates diseases of muscle from diseases of the nerve supply to the muscle.

When the motor neurons supplying a muscle are damaged, either in their cell bodies, the ventral roots, or the peripheral nerve itself, characteristic changes occur in the electromyogram after about three weeks. In contrast to normal muscle, which shows no electrical activity at rest, the denervated muscle fibers generate spontaneous electrical

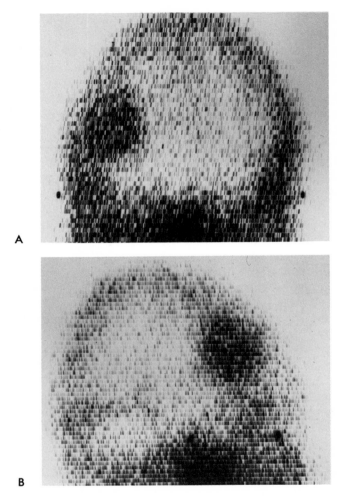

FIG. 37.   Brain scan. (A) Anteroposterior brain scan, showing abnormal uptake of radioisotope in a frontal lobe meningioma. (B) Lateral brain scan, same patient.

potentials called *fibrillations*. These fibrillation potentials are brief diphasic or triphasic waves with amplitudes of 25 to 100 μV. and durations of 0.5 to 1.5 msec. They are the smallest potentials obtainable from muscles, which is not surprising since they are generated from single fibers. Study of appropriate muscles indicate which specific nerve roots, spinal cord segments, or peripheral nerves are damaged (see Tables 3 and 4). Often accompanying these fibrillation potentials in denervated muscle are *fasciculations*, large potentials representing the spontaneous contraction of a *motor unit* (the muscle fibers innervated by a single anterior horn cell) or a portion thereof. Fasciculations are usually visible when the skin over the affected muscle is inspected.

Fasciculations are not always abnormal, however, and a second variety, seen in normal persons, commonly occurs. These are termed *benign fasciculations*. Weakness and atrophy of the muscles are absent in persons with benign fasciculations, and no fibrillations are found on electromyography.

In addition to fibrillations and fasciculations observed when the muscle is at rest, the number of action potentials occurring on voluntary contraction of the muscles is reduced in diseases of the motor neuron, but the size of the potentials remains normal or may be increased. The potentials occurring upon insertion of the needle (insertion potentials) may deviate from the normal pattern.

In diseases of muscles, such as muscular dystrophy or polymyositis, another abnormality of the muscle action potentials, the *myopathic unit*, is observed. Myopathic units are of lower amplitude and duration than normal action potentials, and are usually polyphasic. In muscle disease, the number of action potentials remains normal or nearly so until the disease is advanced. Abnormal irritability of the muscle, manifested by prolonged, repetitive discharges upon insertion of the needle, is also common in muscle diseases, particularly in acute stages.

In addition to these two major disease categories, electromyography has other useful applications. It may provide the earliest evidence of *reinnervation* of a muscle after damage to its nerve. Diseases characterized by rapid fatigability of muscles, such as myasthenia gravis, may be detected by observing the action potentials on the electromyograph during repetitive stimulation of the motor nerve. A fall in amplitude with repeated stimuli is characteristic. Weakness of nonorganic origin often produces a distinctive electromyographic pattern, consisting of bursts of normal-appearing action potentials alternating with little or no activity.

Studies of the *conduction velocities* of motor and sensory nerves offer another aid in the diagnosis of peripheral nerve disease. Stimuli applied to a proximal portion of a motor nerve with a recording electrode inserted into one of the muscles supplied by that nerve provides the basic apparatus for measurement of motor nerve conduction times. Similarly, application of a stimulus to the skin in distal regions of a sensory nerve with a recording electrode proximally over the nerve allows recording of the conduction time of that sensory nerve.

By means of amplifying and time-recording apparatus, the time for the passage of a nerve impulse from the point of stimulus to the point of recording can be measured precisely. When the distance between the stimulating and recording electrode is measured on the patient's limb, the conduction velocity can be calculated. Standard motor and sensory conduction velocities have been determined for several of the peripheral nerves of the body, for example the median, ulnar, and peroneal. Motor velocity for the median and ulnar nerves is 50 to 65 m. per second; that for the peroneal nerve is 40 to 60 m. per second.

Motor and sensory conduction velocity may be reduced in disorders of peripheral nerves. Mild reduction in motor conduction velocity sometimes occurs in chronic diseases of the anterior horn cell or the motor nerve roots, but the sensory conduction velocity remains normal.

The study of certain segments of peripheral nerves is often facilitated by conduction studies. For example, in the carpal tunnel syndrome, a condition resulting from compression of the median nerve as it passes through the wrist into the hand, motor conduction velocity in the median nerve in the forearm is normal, but in that segment of the median nerve crossing the wrist it is reduced.

ELECTROENCEPHALOGRAPHY

The electroencephalogram (EEG) provides a visible record, in the form of wave patterns, of the electrical potentials generated from neuronal activity in the brain. In the usual procedure, 14 or more electrodes are applied to standard locations over the scalp. The electrodes are connected to amplifiers and the potentials recorded on moving paper. Thus, potentials from various areas can be evaluated and compared. Artifacts caused by improper connections, scalp muscle potentials, movement, and other factors may be a source of confusion and must be properly interpreted.

The accepted "normal range" of EEG patterns takes into account the patient's age, state of consciousness, mental state, and routine medications. Deviations from normal patterns may be nonspecific or relatively specific, and their interpretation may differ from one electroencephalographer to another, according to individual criteria. Recordings termed "borderline" by one examiner, for example, may be considered normal by another.

Among the disorders that may induce EEG abnormalities are tumors or other space-occupying intracranial lesions. Tumors in the posterior cranial fossa usually are associated with an abnormal EEG, but the abnormalities are less specific with reference to lateralization and localization. The EEG is abnormal in patients with diffuse metabolic disturbances such as uremia, hepatic coma, drug overdosage, or severe electrolyte and water imbalance, and in infections such as meningitis and encephalitis. The EEG is widely used to aid in the evaluation of patients with convulsive disorders.

The basic rhythm observed in an adult is called the *alpha rhythm* and is maximal posteriorly. It has a frequency of 8½ to 13 Hz. and is present when the patient is relaxed with his eyes closed; it is suppressed when he opens his eyes or concentrates. In more anterior regions a faster rhythm (18 to 30 Hz.) may be seen—the *beta rhythm*. Both alpha and beta rhythms are normally symmetrical bilaterally and have characteristic amplitudes and forms.

If a bright light is flashed in front of the patient's eyes, a rhythmic response that is synchronous with the frequency of the light flashes is recorded from electrodes in the posterior areas of the scalp. This is called "photic driving" and is present normally. Variations from the normal response may indicate brain abnormalities; however, absence of the response is not significant in itself.

The EEG procedure routinely includes a period of hyperventilation by the patient. The resultant decrease in brain carbon dioxide content often induces slowing and increased amplitude of EEG potentials in normal children and young adults. In patients with petit mal epilepsy, the procedure usually evokes a series of three-per-second spike waves and many times an overt seizure; other types of seizures also are induced occasionally.

Induction of sleep during recording may disclose abnormal EEG patterns, such as focal discharges associated with temporal lobe epilepsy, that are not evident when the patient is awake.

The most important abnormalities recorded from adult patients are (1) *delta* waves—2 to 4 Hz.; (2) *spikes*—high-voltage discharges of short duration; (3) *theta* waves—4 to 8 Hz. (not always abnormal); and (4) *asymmetry* of frequency and amplitude from one side to the other (Fig. 38). A small amount of theta and delta activity may occur in normal EEG patterns.

Lesions of many varieties, particularly in acute stages, may suppress the normal alpha rhythm on the side of the lesion. Delta waves are often associated with destruction of brain tissue—infarction, tumor, or abscess—and often are localized over the abnormal area.

Spikes and spike-wave discharges are commonly seen in convulsive

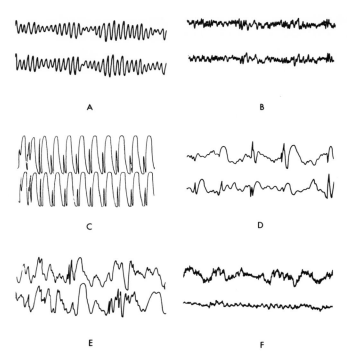

FIG. 38.   Electroencephalograms. (A) Normal alpha rhythm. (B) Beta waves. (C) Three-per-second spike waves in petit mal epilepsy. (D) Spikes and spike waves from temporal lobes in psychomotor epilepsy. (E) Numerous abnormal wave forms in a child with diffuse brain damage ("hypsarrhythmia"). (F) Delta wave focus (*upper portion*) in parietal lobe tumor.

disorders. They may be generalized or focal. In patients with petit mal epilepsy, a three-per-second spike-wave complex is the characteristic abnormality. In patients who have temporal lobe or "psychomotor" seizures, spike complexes occur over the affected temporal lobe. Although the EEG is normal in some patients with grand mal epilepsy, it often shows abnormal paroxysmal features such as high-voltage spikes. In some instances, the EEG may be useful in assessing the effects of treatment. The abolition or reduced frequency of seizures, however, is the major criterion for therapeutic success.

Various metabolic diseases result in diffuse slow waves over the entire brain. In some instances these slow waves are characteristic of the clinical disorder, for example, hepatic coma.

Interpretation of the EEG in children is complicated by the fact that maturation of the brain produces gradual changes in the normal patterns. The basic rhythm is slower, the normal alpha frequency appearing in late childhood. The patient's cooperation is less easily achieved, and thus artifacts appear more frequently.

The EEG is an important test because it is safe and relatively inexpensive and because it is often abnormal in brain diseases. One disadvantage is the difficulty of interpreting borderline or slightly abnormal patterns, since such patterns occur in about 20 percent of the normal population. In the borderline cases, however, serial EEG recordings at selected intervals may yield significant evidence regarding the patient's progress.

INDEX